Topics in Paediatric Psychiatry

Editor: Katharine J. Palmer

last date s

Adis International
Auckland • Buenos Aires • Chester • Hong Kong • Madrid • Milan • Osaka • Paris • Philadelphia • São Paulo • Sydney

Topics in Paediatric Psychiatry

Editor: Katharine J. Palmer

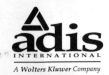

Commercial Manager: Gordon Mallarkey
Publication Manager: Lorna Venter-Lewis
Adis International Limited
Copyright © 2000 Adis International Limited ISBN 0-86471-091-7

Earlier versions of some articles in this book were published in Adis International's peer-reviewed medical journals. The editor has collated the articles and worked with the authors to adapt and update the information for this publication.

Although great care has been taken in compiling and checking the information in this book to ensure it is accurate, the authors, the publisher and their servants or agents shall not be held responsible for the continued currency of the information or from any errors, omissions or inaccuracies arising therefrom, whether arising from negligence or otherwise howsoever or for any consequences arising therefrom.

Printed in Hong Kong.

Foreword

Psychiatric disorders in childhood and adolescence are receiving increasing attention. The impact that these disorders have on the child and his/her family can be great. Rapid diagnosis and appropriate treatment are essential to reduce the long term consequences of the disorders.

This book addresses the diagnosis and treatment of a number of psychiatric disorders that can occur in children and adolescents, including anxiety disorders, bipolar disorder, depression, schizophrenia, attention deficit hyperactivity disorder, and Gilles de la Tourette's syndrome. The focus is on the drug treatment of these conditions, although it is recognised that for many of the disorders, nonpharmacological treatments, such as psychotherapies, family support and educational therapy, play an important role.

The aim of this book is to provide clinicians with current and practical information to assist them in treating psychiatric disorders in their paediatric patients.

Katharine J Palmer
Editor, *CNS Drugs*

August 2000

CNS Drugs is a highly-regarded international medical journal. The journal promotes rational pharmaco-therapy and disease management within the disciplines of clinical psychiatry and neurology by publishing a regular programme of review articles in the subject area.

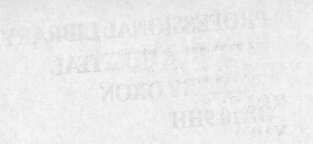

Foreword

Psychiatric disorders in childhood and adolescence are receiving increasing attention. The impact that these disorders have on the child and family can often be great. Rapid diagnosis and appropriate treatment are essential to reduce the long term consequences of the disorder.

This book addresses the diagnosis and treatment of a number of developing disorders that occur in children and adolescents, including anxiety disorders, bipolar disorder, depression, schizophrenia, attention deficit hyperactivity disorder, and Gilles de la Tourette's syndrome. The focus is on the drug treatment of these conditions, although it is recognised that for many of the disorders non-pharmacological treatments, such as psychotherapies, family support and educational therapy, play an important role.

The aim of this book is to provide clinicians with current and practical information to assist them in treating psychiatric disorders in their paediatric patients.

Katharine Johnson
Editor CNS Drugs

August 2002

CNS Drugs is a peer-reviewed international medical journal. The Adis editorial board and independent experts within the discipline determine the development and implementation of the journal's programme of review articles in the subject area.

Topics in Paediatric Psychiatry

Contents

Pharmacological Treatment of Psychiatric Disorders in Children and Adolescents

Focus on Guidelines for the Primary Care Practitioner*

Normand J. Carrey, Doreen M. Wiggins and *Robert P. Milin*

Institute of Mental Health Research and Children's Regional Mental Health Center,
Royal Ottawa Hospital, Ottawa, Ontario, Canada

There is general agreement among epidemiologists that at least 12% of children and adolescents meet criteria for a clinical psychiatric disorder.[1] It is unlikely that specialised health services will be able to deal adequately with this population. Family physicians, paediatricians and school personnel will need to become key elements in the delivery of child mental health services.[2]

The approach taken in this article is to familiarise clinicians with the broad categories of pharmacological agents now available in paediatric psychiatry. The agents reviewed are psychostimulants, antidepressants, anxiolytics, antipsychotics and antimanics. This strictly pharmacological approach has its limitations but also in a sense reflects more closely the symptomatic or behavioural approach to child psychiatric problems. In addition, one drug may have applications across several diagnostic or categorical dimensions.

1. Psychostimulants

There are no cures for attention deficit hyperactivity disorder (ADHD), but successful pharmacological treatment can improve the patient's potential for achievement in academic, family, social and recreation activities. Psychostimulants ameliorate the core presenting symptoms and facilitate other treatments such as school remediation, behavioural therapy and family counselling.[3]

While the use of a psychostimulant may not alter a child's cognition, it may improve the effectiveness of the learning strategies so that distractibility, sustained attention and impulsiveness improve consistently during the performance of cognitive tasks.[4] However, the use of stimulant medication cannot be expected to replace poor learning or social skills that existed before treatment.

Approximately 70% of children diagnosed with ADHD show significant improvement in inattention, hyperactivity and impulsiveness with psychostimulant treatment.[5] Children with a comorbid conduct disorder also appear to respond to treatment with stimulants.[6,7]

Any treatment with medication should be initiated at the lowest dosage possible to minimise

* This article is reprinted unchanged from that published originally in *Drugs* 1996 May; 51: 750-9

potential adverse effects. Increases in dosage should be gradual and titrated individually until optimal effects on behaviour and learning are achieved.[5] Adverse effects are generally dose-dependent, occur at the beginning of treatment and may diminish as the child adjusts to the medication. An adequate medication trial would be 4 to 8 weeks, allowing for titration to optimal dosage.

Methylphenidate and dexamphetamine are the psychostimulants used most frequently. The two drugs are equally effective in therapeutic doses, though dexamphetamine may have more adverse effects than methylphenidate.[8] Treatment effect generally occurs within 1 hour and lasts from 3 to 6 hours, with methylphenidate having a shorter therapeutic effect. Thus, most patients require a second dose around noon. The recommended starting dose is 5mg for methylphenidate and 2.5mg for dexamphetamine. For very young children one-half of this amount is recommended – the dexamphetamine elixir may be simpler to use than a solid dosage form.

The effective daily dose of stimulant medication can vary. An average daily dose of methylphenidate can range from 0.3 to 2.0 mg/kg, and for dexamphetamine from 0.1 to 1.0 mg/kg for children. The average clinical doses therefore are between 10 and 15mg twice daily for methylphenidate and 5 to 10mg twice daily for dexamphetamine. Adolescents may require slightly higher doses, though total daily doses above methylphenidate 60mg or dexamphetamine 40mg are rarely needed.

The long-acting (controlled release; CR) forms of methylphenidate (20mg) and dexamphetamine (spansules) [10 and 15mg] were developed to give sustained behavioural effects. They have a greater delay in the onset of action and for some their effect may not last as long as a second dose of standard medication. Children should be warned not to chew the methylphenidate CR tablet as unpredictably high concentrations of the drug in the blood with toxic effects can result.[9] The CR spansules of dexamphetamine do not present this problem.

Longer-acting stimulants twice daily may be the drug of choice if sustained behavioural effects are needed after school because of social and familial difficulties or organised recreational activities.[10] Clinicians have experimented with combinations of the CR and regular stimulants depending on when during the day the child may exhibit difficulties as a result of inadequate levels of medication. For example, some children may receive regular methylphenidate in the morning in combination with the CR preparation, whereas others may require a noontime addition of regular methylphenidate in addition to their morning CR medication. Alternatively, those receiving standard stimulants could be given a third, smaller dose in the mid-afternoon.

The third available stimulant is pemoline. Like CR methylphenidate and CR dexamphetamine, it has a longer half-life and can be given once a day. Behavioural effects may not be observed for up to 2 weeks, as pemoline may have a small acute effect and a substantial delayed effect,[4] though a recent study suggested that it has an onset of action similar to the other stimulants.[11]

The initial daily dose of pemoline is 18.75mg, with weekly increments of 18.75mg up to 75mg daily (from 0.5 to 3.0 mg/kg/day). Older children may require a slightly higher dosage, up to 112.5mg daily.

Pemoline can cause hepatic toxicity.[12] There have been two reported fatalities but it is not yet established whether the association was causal. Liver function tests are recommended at baseline and repeated at 4- to 6-month intervals for children or adolescents treated and maintained on pemoline.[13,14]

The most common adverse effects of stimulant medications include insomnia, diminished appetite, irritability, gastric upset, headaches and mood alterations. To minimise drug-induced anorexia, medications should be taken with or after meals, and nutritious snacks should be allowed when the child is hungry or at bedtime.[4] Findings on reported growth suppression are contradictory. In one study, reductions of height and weight growth were temporary and minor, and any retardation in the first year was recovered in the second year.[15] In another study, decreases in height and weight percentiles were considered to be significant.[16]

In terms of an initial work-up, height and weight should be checked initially, then every 6 months, and plotted on a standard growth curve. A careful history and physical examination should be done to exclude pre-existing conditions such as cardiac, renal, hepatic or neurological conditions (seizures or tics). At our clinic we do not do routine ECG and additional blood tests unless the physician does it as part of a routine physical examination.

The merit of 'drug holidays' remains unresolved and should be assessed on an individual basis. Those whose symptoms are more noticeable in a school setting may only need to be treated during the school year. Children who manifest significant symptoms in the home environment may not benefit from drug-free holidays.[17] Children should be reassessed on a yearly basis to determine if there still exists a need for the medication.

If there is no need for the child to take the medication on the weekend, the clinician may elect to prescribe it only during the week, although there is no consensus on this practice. Pemoline, because of its longer half-life, must be given continuously throughout the week.

Drug dependence on stimulant medications prescribed for childhood or adolescent hyperactivity has not been demonstrated, as the patient rarely uses stimulant medication to excess.[18] The problem of abuse tends to appear more often in the adults involved with the child being treated,[19] though adolescents with comorbid ADHD and conduct disorder may be at risk for substance abuse. The treating clinician should be aware of the potential for abuse in evaluating the child and family before and during therapy.

The use of stimulant medication for treating ADHD children with tics or Tourette's syndrome remains controversial. Studies have reported on the risk of, or an increase in, tics and tic disorder developing during stimulant treatment.[20,21] Yet Comings and Comings[22] queried the relationship between stimulants and Tourette's syndrome, and recent studies have indicated that psychostimulants may be effective and well tolerated for some children with the syndrome and ADHD.[23-25] Children with comorbid Tourette's syndrome and ADHD are best treated by a specialist.

When serious adverse effects or an incomplete response occur, one stimulant may be substituted for the other. If there is an adequate response but adverse effects are serious, the addition of clonidine may help to alleviate the adverse effect of insomnia as well as to diminish aggression and stimulant-induced physiological rebound. Initial clonidine dosage is 0.025 to 0.05mg at bedtime, with additional doses throughout the day as required to counteract adverse effects or rebound. Older children may require a slightly higher dosage of up to 0.3 mg/day in divided doses.[26] Hypotension is the major adverse effect of clonidine, and blood pressure and pulse should be monitored initially and after each dose increase.

2. Antidepressants

Although widely used in the adult population for the treatment of depression, antidepressants have not been demonstrated to be more effective than placebo in double-blind trials for the treatment of childhood depression.[27] Though data are inconclusive,[27] clinicians have found that on an individual basis antidepressants are effective, especially when psycho-social interventions have failed and there exists a positive family history of depression or anxiety disorders.

In addition, antidepressants have found application in a variety of other childhood disorders such as obsessive-compulsive disorder (OCD), ADHD, enuresis and some other anxiety disorders. Reviewed here are the better known tricyclic antidepressants (TCAs) [e.g. imipramine, clomipramine, desipramine, nortriptyline] and the selective serotonin (S-hydroxytryptamine; S-HT) reuptake inhibitors (SSRIs) [e.g. fluoxetine, fluvoxamine, sertraline and paroxetine].

Imipramine is one of the oldest and most studied antidepressants. It is used for the treatment of depression, and as a second-line treatment for ADHD, anxiety disorders and nocturnal enuresis. Children and young adolescents generally require much lower doses than adults. It is recommended that treatment start with a dosage of 0.5 mg/kg/day, increasing gradually to the lowest dosage that relieves symptoms, or 3.0 mg/kg/day. Some children have responded to higher dosages up to but no more than 5.0 mg/kg/day, but this requires careful monitoring of ECG parameters, and plasma drug concentrations, which should range between 150 and 300 µg/L (combined imipramine and desipramine blood concentrations).[28,29]

Desipramine, the active metabolite of imipramine, has fewer sedative and anticholinergic adverse effects, which makes it better tolerated than the parent drug. More problematic is the purported cardiac toxicity of desipramine, which has been associated with 4 deaths in children.[30] Popper[31] has taken this evidence, and also the finding of lethal toxicity associated with desipramine overdoses, as the basis for the recommendation to choose other anti-depressants to replace desipramine in the treatment of depression or ADHD.

Biederman et al.[32] have done the only study that provides specific data using a 24-hour Holter monitor to assess the cardiac effects of desipramine in children. Findings indicated no drug-associated abnormalities, and the authors concluded that desipramine was a well tolerated medication to administer at therapeutic levels.

Other TCAs, such as nortriptyline[33] and clomipramine,[34] have been shown to be useful in the treatment of various childhood disorders. Clomipramine is effective in the treatment of childhood OCD,[35] because of its serotonergic reuptake blocking properties. Nortriptyline has been found effective in the treatment of ADHD and depression. Clomipramine has the same potency as imipramine while nortriptyline is twice as potent.

For all TCAs, heart rate, blood pressure and ECG intervals need to be recorded at baseline, repeated when the dosage reaches 3.0 mg/kg/day and then with each dose increase afterwards (for imipramine, desipramine and clomipramine) and above 1.5 mg/kg/day for nortriptyline. The following ECG parameters should be followed closely and not exceeded: heart rate >130 beats/min, systolic pressure >130mm Hg, diastolic pressure >85mm Hg, PR interval >200 msec, QRS interval >120 msec (or no more widening than 30% of baseline) and QTc >440 msec.[28,29]

As a class, the TCAs share the following adverse effects that may affect compliance: dry mouth, tremor, sedation (especially imipramine), constipation, weight gain, blurred vision, headaches, and 'jitteriness' or anxiety. For some, daytime sedation can interfere with learning, while anxious children with insomnia may benefit from the sedating effect. With this effect in mind, the clinician should administer the medication throughout the day in divided doses, or all at bedtime. When insomnia is the major symptom we have found that small doses of amitriptyline (10 to 30mg) or trazadone (25 to 50mg) are effective. Weight gain with TCAs can be particularly troublesome with adolescents.

A newer class of agents, the SSRIs, includes fluoxetine, fluvoxamine, sertraline and paroxetine. Individual case studies have indicated the usefulness of fluoxetine in childhood and adolescent depression, but not in a double-blind study.[36] One recent double-blind, placebo-controlled trial has shown that fluoxetine may be effective for depression.[37] Evidence from open trials has indicated that fluoxetine is effective in the treatment of ADHD, especially when it is accompanied by prominent mood symptoms.[38,39] Fluoxetine in a double-blind, crossover trial was found to be useful in the treatment of child and adolescent-onset OCD,[40] though King et al.[41] reported the emergence of self-destructive behaviour in adolescents during fluoxetine treatment.

Daily doses of fluoxetine are not clearly established and may range from 3mg for children up to 20 to 40mg in adolescents. Some children and adolescents may not tolerate daily medication; it can then be given on alternate days. A liquid preparation allows for a more precise titration, and eliminated a rash which accompanied the use of tablets as reported by one of our colleagues (S. Hosenbocus, personal communication).

An open trial of fluvoxamine indicated that it may also be effective in the treatment of adolescent OCD and depression.[42] Experience from our own clinic has shown that fluvoxamine, sertraline and paroxetine are effective in the treatment of individual cases of adolescent depression. The effective dosages for adults are between 50 and 200 mg/day for sertraline and fluvoxamine and from 20 to 40 mg/day for paroxetine and fluoxetine. These dosages should be less for adolescents and children. In fact, Preskorn[43] states that with the SSRIs the starting dose may be the effective dose as well (e.g. in adults, sertraline 50mg or fluoxetine 20mg).

Reported adverse effects with SSRIs include headache, dry mouth and gastrointestinal problems such as nausea, vomiting and diarrhoea. These symptoms usually occur in the first week of treatment, can be transient and resolve with continued treatment. Sexual dysfunction may be frequent, emerge later on in treatment and can be quite alarming – especially to male adolescents. Fluoxetine can induce a behavioural toxicity syndrome of motor restlessness, insomnia, vivid dreams and social disinhibition with possible self-destructive ideation. Popper[31] has noted an amotivational syndrome characterised by apathy (as opposed to an 'I don't care' attitude of depression, it is more an 'I care but it doesn't bother me' attitude), associated with all of the SSRIs. Insomnia is frequently reported with SSRIs and the addition of trazodone in small doses can alleviate this problem.

Finally, two other promising antidepressants should be mentioned. Amfebutamone (bupropion), which blocks dopamine reuptake, has been found to be as effective as methylphenidate in the treatment of ADHD,[44,45] though it may not be available in certain countries. Its main drawback is the higher incidence of seizures. Moclobemide is a reversible monoamine oxidase inhibitor (MAOI) which has the advantage over older MAOIs of not requiring the highly restrictive, low tyramine diet. It has been used in the treatment of childhood ADHD[46] and unpublished reports have indicated that it may be effective in adult ADHD.

For patients who improve significantly on antidepressant treatment it is advisable to continue for up to 6 months before gradually reducing the dosage to determine whether treatment is still needed.[47] Antidepressants should be tapered gradually as flu-like symptoms with gastrointestinal upset and vomiting may occur if medication is discontinued abruptly.

In conclusion, when making the initial choice we recommend the use of SSRIs over the TCAs for the treatment of childhood depression and the use of other tricyclics (nortriptyline or imipramine) rather than desipramine if an antidepressant is used for the treatment of ADHD: if either antidepressant is ineffective or poorly tolerated, desipramine can be used in consultation with a paediatrician or a child psychiatrist. It is worthwhile for the clinician to know the basic differences between the TCAs and the SSRIs in terms of adverse effects, cost and frequency of administration.[43]

3. Anxiolytics

When treating anxiety disorders in children and adolescents, nonpharmacological interventions should always be used initially. Pharmacotherapy should be considered when the symptoms of anxiety are severe, chronic or persistent, and have not responded to psychotherapy or psychosocial interventions. Assessment involves the evaluation of situational factors, family dynamics and school environment. The manipulation of these psychological and environmental factors, before initiating pharmacotherapy, can have a marked effect on outcome in childhood anxiety.

Buspirone is a newly introduced anxiolytic that reportedly causes less sedation, does not interfere with cognitive functioning and has less potential for physiological dependence compared with other anxiolytic medications. Studies in adults have shown it to be effective in treating anxiety disorders, but there have been no controlled trials in children or adolescents. Open studies have indicated that buspirone was effective in controlling hyperactivity and aggression in autistic children,[48] and the symptoms of overanxious adolescents.[49,50] Single-case studies, and an open trial with children and adolescents, also indicated a treatment effect for buspirone either alone or in conjunction with other drugs.[51,52]

Dosage has not been established for children and adolescents, but clinical experience suggests an initial dose of 5mg twice daily titrated weekly by 5mg to a maximum daily dose of 40mg. The patient should be cautioned that therapeutic effect may take 1 to 2 weeks. Reported adverse effects include gastric upset, headaches, restlessness and sedation. These are usually mild and related to increases in dosage. No withdrawal symptoms have been reported at the end of therapy. Because of its slow onset of action, buspirone is not suitable for emergency use or acute situational anxiety: its primary role is in the treatment of long term illness.

Benzodiazepines are frequently used in the treatment of childhood anxiety, but recent conclusive data on efficacy are limited. In addition to their anxiolytic effect, benzodiazepines also have hypnotic, anticonvulsive, disinhibitive, sedative and muscle relaxant properties. While children may have a greater tolerance for the sedative and motor discoordinating effects of benzodiazepines, they may be more susceptible to the disinhibiting effects.[47]

Ultra–short-acting drugs like alprazolam and triazolam are particularly prone to produce rebound syndromes in adults and should probably not be used in children. Clonazepam, which has a longer half-life, has been shown to be effective for panic attacks in children and is probably safer.[53] Dosages vary between 0.5 and 3.0 mg/day.

Indications for the use of benzodiazepines are insomnia, night awakenings, night terrors and somnambulism. Other possible indications are separation anxiety, overanxious disorder and panic attacks.[54] Benzodiazepines should be used with caution in children and adolescents with impulsivity and aggressivity, as disinhibitory effects may aggravate these behaviours.[55] Divided doses 2 or 3 times daily are recommended. Treatment periods should be short term and not exceed 3 to 4 months. Adverse effects include drowsiness, ataxia and behavioural disturbance. Such effects tend to occur early in treatment, are usually dose-related and generally subside with dose reduction and maintenance administration. Withdrawal symptoms and rebound anxiety are possible, and it is important to taper the dosage very gradually at the end of the treatment period. There are no published data on the frequency of any physical or psychologicalal dependence on benzodiazepines in childhood or adolescence.

4. Antipsychotics

The use of antipsychotics is indicated in three general areas: childhood schizophrenia, Tourette's syndrome and behaviour disorders associated with other diagnoses such as severe ADHD, conduct disorder, autism, etc. Most children receiving antipsychotic drugs in clinical practice are not psychotic and the drugs are used in the management of aggression, temper tantrums, stereotypies and hyperactivity.[56] Antipsychotics induce their calming effect through CNS depression. This sedative effect differs from the mechanism of other CNS depressants by producing ataraxia, an arousable anhedonic indifference to the environment, which reduces information flow and hence cognitive overload.[57]

Antipsychotics should be prescribed in low doses and for the shortest possible time (2 to 3 months). Adverse effects include the extrapyramidal symptoms of acute dystonic reactions, akathisia and parkinsonism, while long term CNS complications include tardive dyskinesias.[58,59] The available evidence suggests that children may be more vulnerable to the CNS complications of antipsychotics.

The antipsychotics are generally classified into three categories: (a) the low potency agents (e.g. chlorpromazine and thioridazine); (b) the high potency agents (e.g. haloperidol, thiothixene, pimozide); and (c) the newer atypical antipsychotics (e.g. clozapine and risperidone).

Haloperidol is one of the most widely prescribed high potency antipsychotics. It has been used in the treatment of childhood schizophrenia and Tourette's syndrome, and for aggression associated with autism or mental retardation. The usual dosage is from 0.5 up to 3 mg/day. Cohen and colleagues[60] found that haloperidol was beneficial initially in over 70% of children with Tourette's syndrome, but over the long term only 20 to 30% continued to derive benefit from it. Main adverse effects include fatigue, weight gain, dysphoria, parkinsonism, akathisia and intellectual dulling. These symptoms are of particular concern in school-age children.

Pimozide is a potent antipsychotic similar to haloperidol but less sedating. The usual starting dosage is 1 mg/day, which can be increased to 10 mg/day, with the average daily dose ranging between 2 and 6mg. Because of its long half-life pimozide can be given as a single dose. It has the same indications as haloperidol with a similar adverse effect profile, though it may cause ECG changes such as T wave inversion, U waves, QT interval prolongation and bradycardia.[60] Patients should have an ECG performed at baseline, after dose increases, or at several-month intervals.

Low potency antipsychotics such as chlorpromazine and thioridazine are now rarely used, though they were among the first antipsychotics utilised in the treatment of ADHD. They have been used as an adjunctive treatment to methylphenidate, though clonidine has more recently taken over this role. Low potency antipsychotics are generally indicated in the treatment of aggression in severe conduct-disturbed, autistic or retarded children, either as a single agent or as adjunct therapy. Compared with the high potency antipsychotics they have greater anticholinergic adverse effects with dry mouth, blurred vision, constipation and urinary retention, but fewer extrapyramidal effects. Dosage is initiated at 25 mg/day and may reach a daily maximum of 200 to 300 mg. The regimen is usually 3 times per day, but the full dose may be given at bedtime to enhance sleep and decrease daytime drowsiness.

Clinical experience of atypical antipsychotics is limited and consists mainly of open trials and case studies. In the literature only 20 patients have been treated with risperidone, a potent serotonin, and to a lesser degree dopamine, blocker, after other pharmacological treatments had failed. Simeon and colleagues in seven case studies[61] found it useful for the treatment of schizophrenia, pervasive developmental disorders and severe disruptive disorders. They reported low rates of extrapyramidal effects but some drowsiness at higher dosages. Weight gain was also an adverse effect. Dosage ranged from as low as 0.25 up to 4 mg/day. Mandoki[62] on the other hand reported a higher incidence of extrapyramidal effects in his series of 10 case studies.

Several open case series have been published on the use of clozapine for the treatment of adolescent schizophrenia refractory to other antipsychotics. Clozapine is a strong dopamine D_1 receptor blocker and a weaker D_2 blocker, with a lower incidence of extrapyramidal effects but a higher incidence of anticholinergic effects. Prominent adverse effects are sedation, lowered seizure threshold and blood dyscrasias which necessitate weekly monitoring. Dosages ranged from 100 to 700 mg/day.[63,64]

5. Antimanics

Though lithium is indispensable in treating adults with manic-depressive disorder, it is infrequently used in children and adolescents as the disorder is rarely diagnosed or lithium is of limited efficacy. Carlson[65] recommends using lithium under the following conditions: (a) episodes of mania or depression; (b) history of hypomania and severe depression; (c) severe depression with psychomotor retardation, hypersomnia, psychosis and family history of mood disorder; (d) acute psychotic episode with affective features; and (e) disruptive behaviour disorders with family history of mood disorders, or good response to lithium.

Lithium is utilised more frequently in severe aggression and may be tolerated better than antipsychotics.[66,67] The dosage ranges from 600 to 1200 mg/day in divided doses, and therapeutic concentrations should be between 0.6 and 1.2 mmol/L. Lithium concentrations should be monitored on days 3 and 7 after initiating treatment, weekly for a few weeks and then monthly. Major adverse effects include nausea, vomiting, diarrhoea, fine tremor, increased thirst and urination, and weight gain. Long term adverse effects (6 months to 1 year) are hypothyroidism and structural kidney damage.

Carbamazepine is an anticonvulsant used for treating simple and complex partial seizures, though it may be used in children and adolescents for aggressive or 'explosive' behaviour, and in lithium-resistant mania. Dosage ranges from 200 to 600 mg/day, to produce therapeutic plasma concentrations of 5 to 10 mg/L. Compliance is reduced by the need for weekly blood concentration checks during initial therapy to avoid toxicity and blood dyscrasias such as leucopenia and aplastic anaemia. Recently, the anticonvulsant valproic acid (sodium valproate) has been found to be effective in the control of the acute phase of mania in adolescents and young adults,[68] and the adverse effects may be better tolerated than those of lithium. Generally, the treatment of children and adolescents with these disorders requires referral to a specialist.

6. Conclusion

From a psychopharmacological perspective the range of commercially available drugs, the knowledge about medications, the indications for treatment, and the problems presented by children and adolescents themselves, are rapidly changing. Basic technique, expanding knowledge and the human touch should remain at the centre of child and adolescent treatment.[69]

Medication should always be used to complement other therapies. When pharmacological treatment alleviates the symptoms it allows the clinician to work with the child and family to improve cognitive, behavioural and family dysfunctions. Interventions that assist the mastery of symptoms are important to prevent the return of symptoms after the discontinuation of medication.

Finally, the clinician and psychopharmacologist should be vigilant and sensitive to coercive cultural pressures when drug treatment is either withheld or used too freely in the name of the child's best interest.

References

1. Institute of Medicine. Research on children and adolescents with mental, behavioral and developmental disorders. Washington (DC): National Academy Press, 1989
2. Offord DR, Boyle MH, Fleming JE, et al. Ontario Child Health Study: summary of selected results. Can J Psychiatry 1989; 34: 483-91
3. Koplewicz HS, Williams DT. Psychopharmacological treatment. In: Kestenbaum CJ, Williams DT, editors. Handbook of clinical assessment of children and adolescents. Vol. 2. New York (NY): New York University Press, 1988
4. Dulcan MK. Using psychostimulants to treat behavioral disorders of children and adolescents. J Child Adolesc Psychopharmacol 1990; 1: 7-20
5. Simeon JG, Wiggins DM. Pharmacotherapy of attention-deficit hyperactivity disorder. Can J Psychiatry 1993; 38: 443-8
6. Gadow KD, Nolan EE, Sverd J, et al. Methylphenidate in aggressive-hyperactive boys: I. Effects on peer aggression in public school settings. J Am Acad Child Adolesc Psychiatry 1990; 29: 710-8
7. Kaplan SL, Busner J, Kupietz S, et al. Effects of methylphenidate on adolescents with aggressive conduct disorder and ADHD: a preliminary report. J Am Acad Child Adolesc Psychiatry 1990; 29: 719-23
8. Shekim WO. Diagnosis and treatment of attention deficit and conduct disorders in children and adolescents. In: Simeon JG, Ferguson HB, editors. Treatment strategies in child and adolescent psychiatry. New York (NY): Plenum Press, 1990
9. Ross RB, Licamele WL. Slow-release methylphenidate: problems when children chew tablets. J Clin Psychiatry 1984; 45: 525
10. Pelham WE, Greenslade KE, Vodde-Hamilton M, et al. Relative efficacy of long-acting stimulants on children with attention deficit-hyperactivity disorder: a comparison of standard methylphenidate, sustained-release methylphenidate, sustained-release dextroamphetamine and pemoline. Pediatrics 1990; 86: 226-37
11. Sallee FR, Stiller RL, Perel JM. Pharmacodynamics of pemoline in attention deficit hyperactivity disorder. J Am Acad Child Adolesc Psychiatry 1992; 31: 244-51
12. Nehra A, Mullick F, Ishak KG, et al. Pemoline-associated hepatic injury. Gastroenterol 1990; 99: 1517-9
13. Jaffe SL. Pemoline and liver function [letter]. J Am Acad Child Adolesc Psychiatry 1989; 28: 457-8
14. Greenhill LL. Treatment issues in children with attention-deficit hyperactivity disorder. Psychiatr Ann 1989; 119: 604-13
15. Satterfield JH, Cantwell DP, Schell A, et al. Growth of hyperactive children treated with methylphenidate. Arch Gen Psychiatry 1982; 39: 486-7
16. Mattes J, Gittelman R. Growth of hyperactive children on maintenance methylphenidate. Arch Gen Psychiatry 1983; 30: 317-21
17. Wilens TE, Biederman J. The stimulants. Psychiatr Clin North Am 1992; 15: 191-222
18. Waters BG. Psychopharmacology of the psychiatric disorders of childhood and adolescence. Med J Aust 1990; 152: 32-9
19. Fulton AI, Yates WR. Family abuse of methylphenidate. Am Fam Physician 1988; 38: 143-5
20. Lowe TL, Cohen DJ, Friedhoff AJ, et al. Stimulant medication precipitates Tourette's syndrome. JAMA 1982; 247: 1729-31
21. Calis KA, Grothe DR, Elia J. Attention deficit hyperactivity disorder. Clin Pharmacol 1990; 9: 632-42
22. Comings DE, Comings BG. A controlled study of Tourette syndrome: I. Attention deficit disorder, learning disorders and school problems. Am J Hum Genet 1987; 41: 701-41
23. Konkol RJ, Fischer M, Newby RF. Double-blind, placebo-controlled stimulant trial in children with Tourette's syndrome and attention-deficit hyperactivity disorder. Ann Neurol 1990; 28: 424
24. Gadow KD, Nolan EE, Sverd J. Methylphenidate in hyperactive boys with comorbid tic disorder: II. Short-term behavioral effects in school settings. J Am Acad Child Adolesc Psychiatry 1992; 31: 462-70
25. Rapoport JL, Castellanos FX. Stimulant drug treatment in children with Tourette's syndrome and attention deficit hyperactivity disorder. Clin Neuropharmacol 1992; 15 Suppl. 1: 226A
26. Wilens TE, Biederman J, Spencer T. Clonidine for sleep disturbances associated with attention-deficit hyperactivity disorder. J Am Acad Child Adolesc Psychiatry 1994; 33: 424-6
27. Ambrosini P, Bianchi M, Rabinovitch H, et al. Antidepressant treatments in children and adolescents. J Child Adolesc Psychiatry 1993; 32: 1-6
28. Biederman J, Baldessarini R, Wright V, et al. A double-blind placebo controlled study of desipramine in the treatment of ADD: II. Serum drug levels and cardiovascular findings. J Am Acad Child Adolesc Psychiatry 1989; 28: 903-11
29. Ryan ND. Heterocyclic antidepressants in children and adolescents. J Child Adolesc Psychopharmacol 1990; 1: 2
30. Riddle MA, Geller B, Ryan N. Case study. Another sudden death in a child treated with desipramine. J Am Acad Child Adolesc Psychiatry 1993; 32: 792-7

31. Popper C. Balancing knowledge and judgement: a clinician looks at new developments in child and adolescent psycho-pharmacology. Child Adolesc Clin North Am 1995; 4 (2): 487
32. Biederman J, Baldessarini RJ, Goldblatt A, et al. A naturalistic study of 24-hour electrocardiographic recordings and echocardiographic findings in children and adolescents treated with desipramine. J Am Acad Child Adolesc Psychiatry 1993; 32: 805-13
33. Wilens TE, Biederman J, Geist DE, et al. Nortriptyline in the treatment of ADHD: a chart review of 58 cases. J Am Acad Child Adolesc Psychiatry 1993; 32: 343-9
34. Garfinkel B, Wender P, Sloman L, et al. Tricyclic antidepressant and methylphenidate treatment of attention deficit disorder in children. J Am Acad Child Adolesc Psychiatry 1983; 22: 343-8
35. Flament MF, Rapoport JL, Berg CZ, et al. Clomipramine treatment of childhood obsessive-compulsive disorder: a double-blind controlled study. Arch Gen Psychiatry 1985; 42: 977-83
36. Simeon JG, Ferguson HB, DiNicola VF, et al. Adolescent depression: a placebo-controlled fluoxetine treatment study and follow-up. Prog Neuropsychopharmacol Biol Psychiatry 1990; 14: 791-5
37. Emslie G. The AACAP News. J Am Acad Child Adolesc Psychiatry 1996; Jan-Feb: 15
38. Barrickman L, Noyes R, Kuperman S, et al. Treatment of ADHD with fluoxetine: a preliminary trial. J Am Acad Child Adolesc Psychiatry 1991; 30: 762-7
39. Gammon G, Brown T. Fluoxetine and methylphenidate in combination for treatment of attention deficit disorder and comorbid depressive disorder. J Child Adolesc Psychopharm 1993; 3 (1): 1-10
40. Riddle MA, Scahill L, King RA, et al. Double-blind, crossover trial of fluoxetine and placebo in children and adolescents with obsessive-compulsive disorder. J Am Acad Child Adolesc Psychiatry 1992; 31: 1062-9
41. King RA, Riddle MA, Chapell PB, et al. Emergence of self-destructive phenomena in children and adolescents during fluoxetine treatment. J Am Acad Child Adolesc Psychiatry 1991; 30: 179-86
42. Apter A, Ratzoni G, King RA, et al. Fluvoxamine open-label treatment of adolescent inpatients with obsessive-compulsive disorder or depression. J Am Acad Child Adolesc Psychiatry 1994; 33: 342-8
43. Preskorn SH. Antidepressant drug selection: criteria and options. J Clin Psychiatry 1994; 55 Suppl. A: 6-22
44. Barrickman LL, Perry PJ, Allen AJ, et al. Bupropion versus methylphenidate in the treatment of attention-deficit hyperactivity disorder. J Am Acad Child Adolesc Psychiatry 1995; 34: 649-57
45. Simeon JG, Ferguson HB, Van Wyck Fleet V. Bupropion effects in attention deficit and conduct disorders. Can J Psychiatry 1986; 31: 581-5
46. Trott GE, Friese HJ, Menzel M, et al. Use of moclobemide in children with attention deficit hyperactivity disorder. Psychopharmacol 1992; 106: S134-6
47. Reiter S, Kutcher S, Gardner D. Anxiety disorders in children and adolescents: clinical and related issues in pharmacological treatment. Can J Psychiatry 1992; 37: 432-8
48. Realmuto GL, August GJ, Garfinkel BD. Clinical effect of buspirone in autistic children. J Clin Psychopharmacol 1989; 9: 122-5
49. Kutcher SP, Reiter S, Gardner DM, et al. The pharmacotherapy of anxiety disorders in children and adolescents. Psychiatr Clin North Am 1992; 15: 41-67
50. Kranzler HR. Use of buspirone in an adolescent with overanxious disorder. J Am Acad Child Adolesc Psychiatry 1988; 27: 789-90
51. Simeon JG. Buspirone effects in adolescent psychiatric disorders. Eur Neuropsychopharmacol 1991; 1: 421
52. Simeon JG, Knott VJ, Dubois C, et al. Buspirone therapy of mixed anxiety disorders in childhood and adolescence: a pilot study. J Child Adolesc Psychopharmacol 1994; 4: 159-70
53. Kutcher SP, Mackenzie S. Successful clonazepam treatment of adolescents with panic disorder. J Clin Psychopharmacol 1988; 8: 229
54. Coffey BJ. Anxiolytics for children and adolescents: traditional and new drugs. J Child Adolesc Psychopharmacol 1990; 1: 57-83
55. Simeon JG. Use of anxiolytics in children. Encephale 1993; 9: 71-4
56. Simeon JG. Pediatric psychopharmacology. Can J Psychiatry 1989; 34: 115-22
57. Campbell M, Gonzalez NM, Ernst M, et al. Antipsychotics. In: Werry JS, Aman GA, editors. Practitioner's guide to psychoactive drugs for children and adolescents. New York (NY): Plenum Press, 1993: 269-96
58. Gualtieri CT, Quade D, Hicks RE, et al. Tardive dyskinesia and other clinical consequences of neuroleptic treatment in children and adolescents. Am J Psychiatry 1984; 141: 20-3
59. Sloman L. Use of medication in pervasive developmental disorders. Psych Clin North Am 1991; 14 (1): 165-82
60. Cohen D, Riddle M, Leckman J. Pharmacotherapy of Tourette's disorder. Psychiatr Clin North Am 1992 Mar; 15: 1
61. Simeon JG, Carrey NJ, Wiggins DM, et al. Risperidone effects in treatment-resistant adolescents: preliminary case reports. J Child Adolesc Psychiatry 1995; 5: 69-79
62. Mandoki MW. Risperidone treatment of children and adolescents: increased risk of extrapyramidal side effects? J Child Adolesc Psychopharmacol 1995; 5: 49-67
63. Birmaher B, Baker R, Kapur S, et al. Clozapine for the treatment of adolescents with schizophrenia. J Am Acad Child Adolesc Psychiatry 1992; 31: 160-4
64. Frazier JA, Gordon CT, McKenna K, et al. An open trial of clozapine in 11 adolescents with childhood-onset schizophrenia. J Am Acad Child Adolesc Psychiatry 1994; 33: 658-63
65. Carlson GA. Bipolar disorders in children and adolescents. In: Garfinkel B, Carlson G, Weller E, editors. Psychiatric disorders in children and adolescents. Philadelphia (PA): WB Saunders, 1990
66. Alessi N, Naylor M, Ghaziuddin M, et al. Update on lithium carbonate therapy in children and adolescents. J Am Acad Child Adolesc Psychiatry 1994; 33: 291-304
67. Campbell M, Small AM, Green WH, et al. Behavioral efficacy of haloperidol and lithium carbonate. Arch Gen Psychiatry 1984; 41: 650-6
68. Papatheodorou G, Kutcher S, Katic M, et al. The efficacy and safety of divalproex sodium in the treatment of acute mania in adolescents and young adults: an open clinical trial. J Clin Psychopharmacol 1995 Apr; 15: 110-6
69. Popper C. Introduction: therapeutic empiricism and therapeutic basics. J Child Adolesc Psychopharmacol 1990; 1: 3-5

Correspondence: Dr *Normand J. Carrey,* Royal Ottawa Hospital, 1145 Carling Avenue, Ottawa, Ontario, Canada, K1Z 7K4.

Risk-Benefit Assessment of Pharmacotherapy for Anxiety Disorders in Children and Adolescents

Susan M. Hawkridge and *Dan J. Stein*

Department of Psychiatry, University of Stellenbosch, Tygerberg, South Africa

In recent decades there have been substantial advances in our understanding and management of the anxiety disorders in adults. Epidemiological studies have demonstrated that these disorders are among the most prevalent of the psychiatric disorders.[1] Nosologists have succeeded in separating out 'anxiety neurosis' into various discrete entities with reliable diagnostic criteria. Rigorous controlled trials have led to the introduction of therapies that demonstrate a clear risk-benefit advantage in the drug treatment of these conditions. However, despite the recognition that the anxiety disorders frequently have their onset in childhood or adolescence, there has been relatively little work on anxiety disorders in this population.

Several factors have impeded research in this area. They include rapid changes in diagnostic classifications of childhood and adolescent anxiety disorders; the uncertain reliability of rating instruments for anxiety disorders in this population; and the relatively high comorbidity of other psychiatric disorders, particularly depressive,[2] attention deficit/hyperactivity[2] and substance use disorders,[3] in children with anxiety disorders. Kearney and Silverman draw attention to the fact that even controlled studies in this population should be interpreted with caution, with emphasis on participant selection and attrition, diagnostic criteria and instruments, outcome ratings, comorbidity and psychosocial contextual variables.[4] Suggestions for overcoming some methodological difficulties have been made by Kendall and Flannery-Schroeder[5] and Greenhill et al.[6]

Given the possible severity and chronicity of many childhood and adolescent anxiety disorders,[2] and the relative safety of the newer pharmacotherapeutic agents, there may well be risk-benefit advantages in the use of medication for these conditions. Researchers have gradually begun to gather rigorous data in this area. In a 1995 review, Allen and colleagues found 13 controlled trials of medication for children and adolescents,[7] and some additional trials have been undertaken since that time. Increasingly it is being recognised that ethical concerns about research in this population also need to include consideration of the high personal cost of early onset anxiety disorders and the importance of developing effective treatments.[8]

In this paper we selectively review the literature on pharmacotherapy of anxiety disorders in children and adolescents, focusing in particular on risk-benefit assessment. The review is divided into three sections: the first approaches the subject by focusing on the treatment of the various anxiety disorders seen in children and adolescents, while the second examines the most commonly used medications in these conditions. The third is concerned with risk-benefit assessment and factors influencing choice of drug.

1. Anxiety Disorders in Children and Adolescents

The incidence of clinically significant anxiety in children and adolescents has been found by some authors to be as high as 20% in a non-referred population,[9] far greater than the number of cases that come to the attention of the medical and psychological professions. Factors contributing to this discrepancy may include spontaneous remission, social attitudes concerning the seriousness of emotional, non-disruptive symptoms in children, lack of parental attunement to children's mental states,[10] comparatively low levels of clinician awareness, and the tendency of younger children to somatise symptoms.

Keller et al.[2] found a lifetime history of childhood or adolescent anxiety disorder in 14% of individuals in a community- and clinic-based study (n = 275), with average age of onset of 10 years and a spontaneous remission rate of 34%. A recent twin study in Virginia, US, has documented a 3-month point prevalence of any DSM-III[11] emotional disorder in 8- to 16-year olds of 35.8%, but found that the presence of moderate impairment was limited to 14.2%.[12] However, an increased incidence of interpersonal difficulties, academic impairment, somatic symptoms, poor self-esteem, and depression and suicide in children and adolescents with prominent anxiety symptoms has been described,[9,13] and in an 8-year prospective study, young adults with a history of childhood-onset anxiety disorder were found to be less likely to be living independently than controls with no history of psychiatric illness.[14] Early onset anxiety disorders are among a group of axis I diagnoses found to increase significantly the chance of personality disorder being diagnosed in young adulthood.[15] The importance of effective management of childhood-onset anxiety disorders early in their course may lie in the possibility of prevention of secondary and associated psychopathology.

Establishing reliable diagnostic criteria for childhood and adolescent anxiety disorders is an important step in facilitating their appropriate recognition and treatment. There is a growing trend towards conceptualising the anxiety disorders seen in children as the first onset of disorders usually recognised only later in adults. Of the previously listed Anxiety Disorders of Childhood or Adolescence in the DSM-III-R,[16] only 'separation anxiety disorder' and 're-active attachment disorder' remain as child-specific diagnoses in DSM-IV.[17] 'Overanxious disorder' has been subsumed under 'generalised anxiety disorder', and 'avoidant disorder of childhood or adolescence' now falls under 'social phobia'. The adult criteria have required only minimal modification to accommodate most childhood-onset cases.[17]

While the 'anxious child' has traditionally been treated with psychotherapy alone, the introduction of apparently well tolerated new medications has precipitated a review of the use of psychotherapy as the sole modality of treatment. Although controlled studies of the efficacy of individual, play and family therapies in anxious children are admittedly scarce, there are several studies supporting the use of cognitive-behavioural psychotherapy for anxiety disorders in young patients.[18-21] In addition, a retrospective review of 763 young patients treated at the Anna Freud Centre in London, England, suggested that intensive psychoanalytic therapy over at least 6 months was effective in the treatment of younger children with anxiety disorders, particularly phobic disorders.[22] Most child psychiatrists are likely to agree that the current approach to childhood and adolescent anxiety disorders is ideally multimodal, with attention to family intervention, individual psychotherapy and environmental manipulation, as well as pharmacological treatment where indicated. The use of other or combined modalities is beyond the scope of this review.

1.1 Separation Anxiety Disorder

Separation anxiety disorder in children and adolescents has significant comorbidity with depression,[23] and a history of separation anxiety disorder has been found in up to half of adult study participants with panic disorder and agoraphobia.[24] There is also a strong familial occurrence of these disorders.[25] These findings have led to the hypothesis that the disorders are variants with a common underlying pathophysiology.[24] This offers an explanation for the overlap of the syndromes, and also their documented positive response to the same psychotropic agents, namely the antidepressants.

Early studies, however, focused on the use of benzodiazepines. In an open trial, children with psychiatric disorders were treated with chlordiazepoxide. It was found to be effective in 77% of those with school phobia (n = 50), a heterogeneous group in whom separation anxiety disorder is commonly the primary diagnosis.[26] A smaller open-label study of 9 children with school phobia (again with prominent symptoms of separation anxiety) found chlordiazepoxide 10 to 30mg daily to be a useful adjunct to psychotherapy, enabling 8 of the children to return to school within 2 weeks without serious discomfort.[27]

There have been five placebo-controlled studies of the efficacy of tricyclic antidepressants (TCAs) in separation anxiety and/or school refusal. An early study using imipramine 100 to 200 mg/day (mean = 152 mg/day) plus behavioural treatment for 6 weeks showed an 81% return to school (n = 16), which was significantly better than a 47% return rate in the group receiving placebo plus behavioural treatment (n = 19). Of interest is that at 3 weeks there was still no difference between the drug group and the placebo group in terms of return to school.[28] However, an attempt to replicate this study in children who had not responded to 4 weeks of behavioural treatment (21 of 45), failed to show any superiority of imipramine over placebo, with an overall improvement rate of 50% in both groups. [29] It should be noted that the number of participants is small in this last study, making interpretation of the results difficult. Similarly, in a 12-week double-blind trial comparing clomipramine (40 to 75mg/day) with placebo in 51 children and adolescents with school refusal (87% with separation anxiety), clomipramine was not found to be superior to placebo in alleviating anxiety/depression symptoms or facilitating a return to school.[30] It is possible that higher doses of clomipramine might have been more effective.

An 8-week placebo-controlled trial of cognitive-behavioural therapy with imipramine (average dosage 182.3 mg/day) or placebo in 47 adolescents with school refusal showed a significantly greater and more rapid improvement in school attendance in those receiving imipramine. However, all participants had major depressive disorder and an anxiety disorder, making interpretation of these data in this context difficult.[31]

The high potency benzodiazepine clonazepam, given as a daily dose of 0.5 to 3mg, was found to be effective in 3 children with separation anxiety and panic-like symptoms who had not responded adequately to other forms of therapy, including imipramine (n = 2) and alprazolam (n = 1).[32] Nevertheless, results from a controlled study were more ambiguous. An 8-week double-blind, crossover trial of clonazepam (up to 2 mg/day) versus placebo was carried out involving 12 children with anxiety disorders, 11 of whom had separation anxiety disorder and 10 of whom had more than one diagnosis, including generalised anxiety disorder, oppositional defiant disorder, avoidant disorder/social phobia and attention deficit/hyperactivity disorder. At the end of the study, 50% of those who completed the trial no longer met the criteria for an anxiety disorder, but there was no significant improvement relative to baseline for either group according to the Brief Psychiatric Rating Scale (BRPS) or Clinical

Global Impression (CGI) scale. The authors suggested that a longer duration of treatment may be required for improvement.[33]

An open trial of imipramine (mean dosage = 135 mg/day) versus alprazolam (mean dosage = 1.43 mg/day) in 17 children refusing to attend school showed a 50 and 55% return to school respectively,[34] but a subsequent controlled trial of alprazolam (mean dosage = 1.82 mg/day) versus imipramine (mean dosage = 164 mg/day) versus placebo in 24 different children refusing to attend school did not find significant intergroup differences in outcome. However, at week 8 there were significantly greater reductions in both anxiety and depression symptoms for the children taking imipramine or alprazolam, with alprazolam somewhat superior to imipramine. Six children completed the study in each group, and all except one placebo group participant returned to school with improved attendance.[34] Both studies included a high percentage of individuals with comorbid depression.

In an open label study of 21 children, 15 of whom had separation anxiety disorder in addition to overanxious disorder and/or social phobia, fluoxetine (mean dosage 25.7 mg/day) was found to be effective in achieving a marked to moderate reduction in anxiety symptoms in 81%.[35] Initial dosages were low (10mg three times per week), and therapeutic effect was noted to begin after 6 to 8 weeks of drug treatment. The medication was well tolerated. In another open study, 10 of 10 patients with separation anxiety disorder responded to treatment with fluoxetine (mean dosages: children = 24 mg/day; adolescents = 40 mg/day).[36]

In summary, while there is only one early controlled trial which clearly points to the efficacy of medication for separation anxiety disorder, it seems clear that benzodiazepines and TCAs may be useful in some children. Given their relative safety and promising efficacy, the use of selective serotonin (5-hydroxytryptamine; 5-HT) reuptake inhibitors (SSRIs) should also be considered. Further controlled studies of these agents in larger diagnostically distinct groups are necessary to establish efficacy in this disorder.

1.2 Panic Disorder with or without Agoraphobia

Data on the treatment of childhood and adolescent panic disorder are predominantly limited to case reports and small open trials. TCAs (imipramine and desipramine), for example, were found to be effective in 3 adolescents[37] and in an 8-year-old boy[38] with panic disorder. An earlier report described 3 children (aged 8 to 13 years) whose panic disorder with agoraphobia responded to imipramine (75 to 125 mg/day) with or without alprazolam 1mg twice daily.[39]

Similarly, clonazepam (0.5 to 3 mg/day) has been described as effective in 3 prepubertal children with panic-like symptoms.[32] A report of 4 adolescents with panic disorder showed clonazepam 0.5mg twice daily to result in a decrease of mean panic attack frequency from 3 per week to 0.25 per week. There was also a decrease in the mean anxiety score, as measured on the Hamilton Anxiety Rating Scale (HARS), from 32 to 5.7 over 2 weeks of treatment.[40]

In addition, results of a double-blind study of 12 adolescents with panic disorder treated with clonazepam showed that 80% of patients receiving clonazepam achieved a moderate or marked improvement on the CGI scale versus 20% of the patients receiving placebo. The mean panic attack frequency fell from 2 to 0.5 per week in the group receiving clonazepam and from 2 to 1.8 per week in the placebo group. Mean HARS score fell from 25 to 10 in the group receiving clonazepam, and from 29 to 21 in the placebo group.[41]

Propanolol has been reported to be useful in the treatment of paediatric hyperventilation syndrome, a possible panic disorder variant. Of 14 patients in an open-label series, 13 responded positively to propanolol 30 to 60 mg/day, but relapse occurred within 5 days of cessation of treatment in 8 of the 13 responders.[42]

There are clearly inadequate controlled data to indicate clear efficacy of any medication in panic disorder in children, but the one controlled trial suggests that clonazepam is an effective treatment in adolescents. In adults with panic disorder, the efficacy of SSRIs is well established, although it appears that patients with panic disorder are exquisitely sensitive to adverse effects and initial dosage needs to be very low with gradual upward titration.[43] The addition of a high potency benzodiazepine in the initial stages of treatment may be useful but the potential for dependency warrants caution. Additional research is necessary before clinical guidelines for younger patients can be given with certainty.

1.3 Social Phobia

Black and Uhde[44] described the case of a 12-year-old patient with elective mutism and social phobia who did not respond to 10 weeks of desipramine 200 mg/day, but did respond to fluoxetine 20 mg/day within 4 weeks. Subsequently, an open study of fluoxetine for elective mutism with comorbid overanxious disorder or social phobia in 21 children found that the response was better in those patients under 10 years of age.[45] In an open trial of fluoxetine in the treatment of social phobia, 8 of 10 children and adolescents showed an improvement, with younger patients who had only one anxiety disorder diagnosed tending to respond to lower dosages than those with more than one anxiety disorder (i.e. 0.49 versus 0.8 mg/kg/day).[36]

However, a 12-week, placebo-controlled study of fluoxetine 12 to 27 mg/day in the treatment of 15 children and adolescents with selective mutism and social phobia or avoidant disorder showed only one significant difference: the parents' rating of global improvement and mutism improvement was greater in those individuals receiving fluoxetine.[46] Campbell and Cueva[47] have questioned the significance of this result, as selective mutism is characteristically not prominent in the home environment.

A 6.5-year-old girl with selective mutism, oppositional defiant disorder and mild obsessive-compulsive behaviour treated with fluvoxamine 50 to 100 mg/day showed resolution of selective mutism, but persistence of other symptoms and the emergence of hypomanic behaviour as a dose-limiting adverse effect.[48] A review of 7 patients aged 7 to 18 years with the primary diagnosis of generalised social phobia who were treated with paroxetine, nefazodone or sertraline reported that all three agents were effective and well tolerated.[49] There is one case report of the successful use of buspirone 20 mg/day in an adolescent with social phobia complicating schizotypal/schizoid personality disorder.[50]

A double-blind, placebo-controlled trial over 4 weeks of alprazolam 0.5 to 3.5 mg/day in the treatment of 30 children and adolescents with avoidant or overanxious disorder showed a slightly greater improvement in those with avoidant disorder treated with alprazolam, but this result failed to reach statistical significance. [51]

In adults, monoamine oxidase inhibitors (MAOIs) such as phenelzine [52] have been shown to be effective in the treatment of generalised social phobia. These agents have not been well studied in children. In one case report, a 7-year-old girl with selective mutism was successfully treated with phenelzine 60 mg/day.[53] A 6-year-old girl with selective mutism and Tourette's syndrome responded partially to fluoxetine 20 mg/day but obtained full remission of symptoms when haloperidol 0.5mg twice daily for tics was added and fluoxetine was increased to 30 mg/day.[54]

Limited social phobia or performance anxiety has been successfully treated with a single dose of a β-blocker given prior to the anticipated stressor (e.g. exam, performance, etc.) in the vast majority of studies in adults.[55] In one study of students, oxprenolol proved more effective than diazepam in reducing anxiety and improving examination performance.[56] However, no specific data on the use of these agents for performance anxiety in children or adolescents were found in the literature.

Given the increasing successful use of SSRIs in adults with social phobia[57,58] and the possibility that these agents may be helpful in the treatment of social phobia symptoms in children, it seems reasonable to consider their use in this somewhat resistant condition. Once again, this is a field in which additional controlled trials are necessary.

1.4 Simple Phobia

To our knowledge, no controlled studies on the pharmacotherapy of simple phobia have been conducted to date. Behavioural/cognitive-behavioural therapy remains the treatment of choice,[59] although there are indications that intensive psychoanalytical therapy may also be effective. [22] Reports of the successful treatment of an 11-year-old boy with a specific phobia of storms with fluvoxamine 50 mg/day[60] and a 2.5-year-old girl with specific phobia and panic attacks with fluoxetine 5 mg/day[61] suggest that, when behavioural therapy is impractical, SSRIs may be a useful alternative. Given the high incidence of specific phobia in children, further research in this area is warranted.

1.5 Obsessive-Compulsive Disorder

The finding that serotonin reuptake inhibitors were useful in adults with obsessive-compulsive disorder (OCD) encouraged trials of these agents in children and adolescents. Clomipramine 140 to 200 mg/day[62-64] and fluoxetine 20 mg/day[65] have been established as well tolerated and superior to placebo in the treatment of OCD in children and adolescents in controlled trials. A retrospective review of 20 children and 18 adolescents treated with fluoxetine for OCD showed similar responses in both age groups at similar bodyweight-adjusted dosages (mean dosage 50 mg/day).[66] Fluvoxamine was found to be effective and well tolerated in an open trial,[67] as were sertraline[68] and citalopram.[69] This has been now been confirmed for fluvoxamine and sertraline in placebo-controlled trials.[70-72] A large (n = 187) randomised, double-blind, placebo-controlled trial confirmed the safety and efficacy of sertraline titrated to a maximum of 200 mg/day (average dosage 167 mg/day) in the treatment of OCD in children and adolescents.[72] The superiority of sertraline over placebo emerged at week 3 of the study. Paroxetine (10 to 60 mg/day) was found to be effective in the treatment of 20 paediatric outpatients with OCD in an open-label study.[73]

Thus, despite as yet inadequate data concerning their long term use, SSRIs may now be considered the pharmacotherapy of choice in younger patients with OCD.

The combination of SSRI and clomipramine was administered to 7 patients aged 9 to 23 years with OCD resistant to monotherapy, and resulted in symptomatic improvement in all 7.[74] However, 5 of the 7 participants developed adverse effects, in particular cardiovascular abnormalities. SSRIs can increase the plasma concentration of TCAs and meticulous monitoring appears warranted if such combinations are used.

It is likely that pharmacotherapy in both children and adults needs to be maintained for some time, as relapse may follow discontinuation of medication.[75] While it is probable that combining medication with behaviour therapy allows earlier or more successful tapering of medication, this remains to be proven in controlled trials. Cognitive behavioural therapy has been shown to be an effective treatment for the disorder, alone or in combination with drug therapy.[76] Further long term studies are needed, as well as studies of pharmacotherapy versus psychotherapy versus combination therapy.

In adults with OCD, the presence of comorbid tics has been associated with relative failure to respond to serotonin reuptake inhibitors.[77] Similarly, 11 children with comorbid Tourette's syndrome and obsessive-compulsive symptoms did not show a significantly better response to fluoxetine than to placebo.[78] However, in a retrospective study, 76% of 30 patients with Tourette's syndrome and comorbid obsessive-compulsive behaviours responded to fluoxetine 20 to 40 mg/day.[79] Such comorbidity in children and adolescents may require combined therapy with both serotonin reuptake inhibitors and dopamine blockers.[80]

A subgroup of children has been identified who develop OCD (with or without a movement disorder) following infection with group A β-haemolytic streptococcus. Immunomodulatory therapies and antibiotics may prove to be effective, both acutely and in long term maintenance and prophylaxis.[81]

The pharmacotherapy of disorders postulated to fall on a spectrum of OCD-related disorders is not well studied in children and adolescents. Further attention to the use of medication in disorders such as body dysmorphic disorder, trichotillomania and possibly related conditions in this age group is warranted.

1.6 Post-Traumatic Stress Disorder

A report of the use of propanolol to treat agitation in 11 children with post-traumatic stress disorder (PTSD) following abuse indicated a reduction in symptoms on this medication.[82] There are also some promising preliminary data on the use of clonidine in the treatment of severe PTSD in 7 preschool children.[83]

Treatment recommendations are not possible, given the current lack of published data on pharmacotherapy in young patients with PTSD.[84] Although the SSRIs are receiving increased attention in adults with PTSD,[85] there is relatively little reported on their use in children with this condition. An open trial of citalopram in adolescents with PTSD, currently in press, suggests that this agent may be effective.[85a] In view of the existing data and the relative safety of the SSRIs in clinical practice they should be considered in children and adolescents with PTSD.

1.7 Generalised Anxiety Disorder

Previously referred to as overanxious disorder of childhood, this disorder is one of the more common anxiety disorders in children, with the incidence in a community study ranging from 8.6% in 8-year-olds to 17.1% in 17-year-olds.[9] Despite this, and possibly because it is often comorbid with other anxiety disorders (>50%), there are few studies of the specific pharmacotherapy of this condition.

An 11-week, single-blind study of alprazolam 0.5 to 1.5 mg/day in 12 children and adolescents with overanxious and/or avoidant disorder showed a significant improvement in CGI, and anxiety and depression ratings during the active phase of treatment, but nonresponse and relapse during the placebo phases.[86] However, a subsequent 6-week, double-blind, placebo-controlled study using a larger sample (n = 30) showed no significant superiority of alprazolam 0.5 to 3.5 mg/day over placebo. [51]

In an open trial of fluoxetine 10 to 60 mg/day in 21 children and adolescents with overanxious disorder, separation anxiety disorder and/or avoidant disorder, and excluding OCD and panic disorder, there was moderate to marked improvement in 81% after 6 to 8 weeks.[35] There are no published controlled trials of antidepressants in children and adolescents with generalised anxiety disorder. However, these agents may be useful in at least some of these patients.

A controlled study of hydroxyzine versus buspirone versus placebo in adults with generalised anxiety disorder suggests that hydroxyzine may show a slight clinical advantage in the treatment of this disorder in adults.[87] Since this drug is still used by some clinicians for the acute management of anxiety in children despite a lack of supportive data, a troublesome adverse effect profile and the existence of more specific alternatives, controlled research in younger patients appears desirable.

A single case report of an adolescent treated with buspirone 7.5 to 15 mg/day, started after adverse effects had limited the use of desipramine 125 mg/day, suggests that this agent might be a useful treatment for generalised anxiety disorder in adolescents.[88] Furthermore, an open label study of adolescents with generalised anxiety disorder/overanxious disorder showed significant reduction of anxiety symptoms after 6 weeks of buspirone 15 to 30 mg/day.[41] Given the efficacy of buspirone in adults with generalised anxiety disorder and its apparently favourable adverse effect profile, this agent appears to be a useful choice in children and adolescents with this disorder and deserves further study in controlled trials.

In summary, there is, at present, no incontrovertible evidence supporting the use of benzodiazepines, antidepressants or buspirone in the treatment of generalised anxiety disorder in young patients. Controlled trials are imperative, given the frequency of the disorder and the widespread empirical use of such medications in its treatment.

1.8 Anxiety Disorder due to Substance Use or to General Medical Conditions

Anxiety disorder due to substances or to general medical conditions is not uncommon in certain clinical settings. Nevertheless, these disorders have not been well researched. In clinical practice, treatment involves addressing the underlying substance use disorder or general medical condition and the short term use of benzodiazepines where necessary. Where prescription medication at therapeutic doses is the cause, review of drug choice is indicated. For example, a recent report cites three cases of separation anxiety developing as an adverse effect of treatment with risperidone. Two of these patients had a childhood history of separation anxiety disorder. Symptoms resolved on withdrawal of risperidone, and two of the boys were subsequently treated with olanzapine without recurrence of separation anxiety symptoms.[89]

Serious medical conditions in children may cause severe anxiety that warrants independent attention. Hanna et al.[90] describe the successful treatment of a 4-year-old boy with laryngomalacia and pharyngeal dysphagia who experienced extreme anxiety associated with eating as well as separation and social anxiety. Buspirone in a gradually increasing dosage up to 12.5 mg/day resulted in resolution of symptoms, with relapse on discontinuation.[90]

1.9 Anxiety Symptoms in Other Psychiatric Disorders

There are several case reports and open trials suggesting that serotonin reuptake inhibitors may be beneficial in the treatment of obsessive-compulsive behaviours or anxiety symptoms in children and adults with developmental disorders.[91-96] In a 10-week, double-blind, placebo-controlled trial, clomipramine (mean dosage = 152 mg/day) was found to be superior to desipramine (mean dosage = 127 mg/day) and placebo in the treatment of stereotypies and obsessive-compulsive symptoms in 24 autistic children (aged 6 to 18 years).[97] Fluvoxamine was found to be similarly effective in a controlled study of autistic adults.[98] Propanolol[99] and imipramine[100] have also been reported as beneficial in single case reports. More recently, a reduction in anxiety symptoms, among others, was reported in 8 children, adolescents and adults who had pervasive developmental disorder and were treated with olanzapine (mean dosage 7.8 mg/day) for 12 weeks.[101]

2. Drugs Used to Treat Anxiety in Children: Adverse Effects and Efficacy

2.1 Benzodiazepines

Benzodiazepines have long been established as useful in decreasing the symptoms of anxiety.[26,102] The literature concerning adults has examined the risk of tolerance, dependency and abuse. Additional important adverse effects that require consideration in children and adolescents include cognitive impairment, disinhibition, and depression.[26]

For example, in an early open trial of chlordiazepoxide 30 to 110 mg/day in divided doses in 130 children with various diagnoses,[26] 41% were rated as having a 'good' to 'excellent' response. Drowsiness and dizziness occurred in about 20%, although this was transient and responsive to dose reduction in most. Depression necessitated withdrawal of the medication in 2 patients. A 'paradoxical reaction' of hyperactivity, rage and dyscontrol occurred in 10%. Of these 13 children, 5 had abnormal electroencephalograms, suggesting that this may be a risk factor for adverse behavioural reactions to benzodiazepines. In a more recent report, 3 of 4 children who developed behavioural disinhibition when treated with clonazepam had underlying structural brain damage, thus supporting this hypothesis.[103]

Similar adverse events have been reported in controlled trials of benzodiazepines in children and adolescents. In a double-blind study of clonazepam in 12 adolescents with panic disorder, minimal adverse effects were reported, most commonly transient mild drowsiness, but increasing irritability and restlessness caused 1 person to withdraw from the study.[41] In a placebo-controlled study of clonazepam at a dosage of up to 2 mg/day in 12 children with anxiety disorders (11/12 had separation anxiety disorder and 10/12 had more than one diagnosis), mild to severe adverse effects (drowsiness, irritability/lability and oppositional behaviour) were experienced by 83% of those receiving clonazepam and 58% of those receiving placebo, the difference not reaching significant levels. However, 3 boys had to be withdrawn from the trial during the active phase owing to serious disinhibition with marked irritability, tantrums and aggressive behaviour. The authors suggested that the rather steep induction rate (0.25mg every 3 days to 1mg then every 2 days to 2mg) may have contributed to the adverse effects.[33] Irritability and behavioural outbursts have been reported in adolescents treated with clonazepam[104] and toxicity with psychotic symptoms has been reported in 2 children.[105]

Recent findings on the effect of some benzodiazepines on the immune system raise concerns about the potential dangers of these drugs, particularly in immune-compromised individuals.[106] However, further research in this area is needed before definitive conclusions can be reached.

In children and adolescents, as in adults, withdrawal symptoms can be severe, and gradual tapering of dosage is essential.[107]

In summary, while the benzodiazepines may be useful for the short term treatment of anxiety symptoms in some children and adolescents, the potential for dependence and other adverse effects makes them less than ideal agents. Benzodiazepines should therefore be used with caution and for as short a time as possible.

2.2 Tricyclic Antidepressants

The emergence of self-destructive behaviour in a child with Tourette's syndrome and OCD treated with clomipramine 20 to 50 mg/day,[108] and paranoid and aggressive behaviour in 2 adolescents with OCD treated with clomipramine 75 to 200 mg/day,[109] has been reported.

The potentially dangerous cardiovascular adverse effects of imipramine and desipramine, particularly at high doses, have long been a subject of concern to clinicians. Increased heart rate,[110] PR interval prolongation, QTc lengthening and QRS widening[111] have all been re-ported in children and adolescents. Of 16 children aged 7 to 12 years, 3 developed first degree atrioventricular block while receiving imipramine 50 to 159 mg/day, and plasma concentra-tions above 225 μg/L were consistently shown to slow intracardiac conduction.[112] In a series, 6 of 30 patients aged 6 to 17 years developed a right bundle branch block–type conduction defect while receiving desipramine at a dosage of up to 5 mg/kg/day (mean = 2.7) and 1 developed an atrioventricular block.[111] Desipramine also significantly reduces heart rate variability in children, adolescents and adults.[113,114] A study, which included 4 children and 5 adolescents, of cardiovascular changes during exercise in patients receiving desipramine (mean dosage 3 mg/kg/day) confirmed this effect, but showed only modest medication effects on blood pressure.[115]

In a review of the pre- and intratreatment electrocardiograms of 39 children given imipra-mine or desipramine, 11 showed an increase of 0.02 seconds or more in the PR interval, and a new first degree atrioventricular block developed in 2 participants. Those with pretreatment conduction abnormalities were more likely to develop an increase in the PR interval of 0.02 seconds or more. Intratreatment abnormalities did not correlate with the choice or dosage of drug and none of the participants showed any clinical adverse cardiovascular responses.[116]

A series of 7 younger patients treated with a combination of SSRIs and clomipramine showed two of the participants developing QTc interval prolongation and two developing tachycardia.[74] The concurrent use of these medications may increase the risk of cardiovascular adverse effects, as SSRIs can increase the plasma concentrations of TCAs.

Particular caution seems warranted when treating anxious children who are concurrently receiving medication for medical conditions. In a series of 28 anxious and/or depressed chil-dren with asthma who were taking an average of 5 medications for this condition as well as TCAs, 4 patients developed significant cardiovascular adverse effects.[117]

The most disturbing adverse event associated with treatment with TCAs is the intermittent reporting of sudden death in young children taking these drugs, often at relatively low dosages.[118] It remains unclear whether these deaths reflect pre-existing cardiac dysfunction or are a direct consequence of pharmacotherapy with these agents.[119] Nevertheless, given these findings, the use of TCAs, in particular desipramine, in children and adolescents seems warranted only when alternatives are not available, psychopathology is severe and there is relatively good expectation of their efficacy. When the decision to use these agents is made, careful electrocardiogram monitoring is required. Late onset electrocardiographic changes during long term maintenance treatment have been reported.[120]

Cohen and colleagues failed to find any contribution of age or gender to desipramine clearance in 173 children and adolescents.[121] However, wide interpatient variability in desi-pramine clearance rates was confirmed, and the authors postulate that these differences may be genetically determined. The lethality of TCAs in overdose is well documented and reliable adult supervision of medication should be assured before they are prescribed.

2.3 Selective Serotonin Reuptake Inhibitors

In a study of 24 children and adolescents with OCD or depression treated with fluoxetine 20 to 40 mg/day, Riddle et al.[122] found a 50% incidence of agitation, motor restlessness and sleep disturbance. A second report in the same year from the same group of researchers detailed the emergence of self-destructive behaviour in 6 patients aged 10 to 17 years who were treated with fluoxetine for OCD.[123] Of these patients, 4 required hospitalisation for their symptoms. Several hypotheses have been advanced in explanation of these adverse effects – the behaviour may emerge as a result of the activation of specific mechanisms in vulnerable individuals, possibly producing a type of frontal lobe disinhibition syndrome,[124] or the agitation may be secondary to akathisia or the drug has a specific effect on the regulation of aggression.[123] An open trial of the effect of SSRIs on aggressive behaviour in adolescents found that patients displayed more verbal aggression, physical aggression towards objects and physical aggression towards self when on medication than when off.[125]

Additional troublesome adverse effects of the SSRIs emerged in a series of 20 adolescents treated with fluvoxamine for OCD or depression and included hyperactive behaviour, excitement and increased anxiety in 3 patients (severe in 1), hypomania in 1, dermatitis in 3, nausea in 3, drowsiness in 2, and insomnia in 4.[67] March et al.[72] reported insomnia (37%), nausea (17%), agitation (13%) and tremor (7%) in a large series of children and adolescents treated for OCD with sertraline (mean dosage 167 mg/day). 13% of 92 patients discontinued treatment as a result of adverse events. Similar findings were reported in a 10-week open-label study of sertraline (mean dosage 127.2 mg/day) in the treatment of 53 depressed adolescents, of whom one discontinued treatment because of akathisia.[126]

Sertraline used in the treatment of anxiety symptoms in autistic children caused deterioration in behaviour at higher dosages in 2 of 9 children,[94] but in a larger study the major adverse effect reported was gastric discomfort.[68] More serious adverse effects reported include hallucinations and delirium (1 each), but these appear to have been limited to 2 debilitated girls with anorexia nervosa.[67] Sporadic case reports of mania or hypomania[48,127,128] and extrapyramidal symptoms[129,130] as complications of treatment with SSRIs in adolescence have appeared.

Paroxetine (10 to 60 mg/day) in the treatment of 20 paediatric outpatients with OCD was reported to cause hyperactivity/behavioural disinhibition (30%), headache (25%), insomnia (15%) and anxiety (10%), among adverse effects.[73] Behavioural disinhibition necessitated dosage reduction in 3 patients under the age of 10 years. An open trial of paroxetine (mean dosage 16.22 mg/day) in 45 depressed children under the age of 14 reported only transient gastrointestinal adverse effects, which were successfully managed by temporary dosage reduction.[131]

In an open trial of fluoxetine over 10 months, 21 children and adolescents with overanxious disorder, social phobia or separation anxiety disorder were treated with a mean dosage of 27.5 mg/day, starting with 10mg every second day. Reported adverse effects included insomnia (3 cases), nausea (3 cases), stomach ache, mild headache and anorexia (1 each). There were no reports of agitation, hypomanic behaviour or suicidal ideation. 81% showed moderate to marked improvement.[35] Similar adverse effects were recorded in an earlier study[132] and in a later open trial.[36]

These contradictory findings may be related to different initial doses used in the studies. It is possible that low initial doses with slow increments may avoid the behavioural adverse effects seen in earlier studies. The disparate findings may also reflect differences in the underlying neurobiology of the different disorders studied by these groups.

In addition, there is the potential for sexual dysfunction, an adverse effect of the SSRIs well known in adults,[133] to limit compliance in older adolescents, and one case of hypersexuality has been reported in a 15-year-old boy.[134] Memory impairment has been described as a rare adverse effect of fluoxetine in adults, and there is at least one report of similar difficulties complicating fluoxetine treatment of an adolescent.[135]

A report of increased blood pressure (>10mm Hg) and pulse rate (>10) in more than 50% of children aged 4 to 12 years receiving fluoxetine (mean dosage = 19 mg/day), sertraline (mean dosage = 75 mg/day) or imipramine (mean dosage = 86 mg/day) with no significant intergroup differences raised concerns about possible cardiovascular adverse effects of the SSRIs.[136] However, a study of 92 children and adolescents treated with sertraline (average dosage 167 mg/day) for OCD found no clinically significant cardiovascular adverse effects as measured by electrocardiogram, blood pressure and pulse.[137] A recent report has highlighted the possibility of an interaction between stimulant drugs and sertraline resulting in a serious cardiovascular adverse effect (atrioventricular nodal re-entrant tachycardia).[138] A review of paediatric paroxetine overdoses suggests that this agent is unlikely to cause toxic effects even in very young children when ingested alone.[139]

There is also concern about a discontinuation syndrome following use of SSRIs in adults.[140] There are no available data in this regard for children and adolescents, but there is no reason to believe that they are exempt from this phenomenon. If it does occur in the younger patient, it may complicate termination of treatment with these agents.

Certainly, caution is always required when using antidepressants in children and adolescents. Furthermore, studies to date have primarily focused on fluoxetine, fluvoxamine and sertraline, and controlled data on other SSRIs are needed. Nevertheless, in clinical practice the largely favourable adverse effect profile of these agents makes them a useful choice, and there is increasing evidence of their efficacy in a number of childhood and adolescent anxiety disorders. Further studies with larger samples are needed to establish firm guidelines for their use.

2.4 Other Agents

Buspirone is a serpotonin 5-HT_{1A} receptor agonist that has been shown to be effective for generalised anxiety disorder in adults and that appears to have an acceptable adverse effect profile. Furthermore, preliminary data on the safety of this agent in adolescents and children with generalised anxiety disorder are favourable.[141,90] However, in an open-label study of buspirone (up to 50 mg/day) in 25 prepubertal children with anxiety and aggression, 6 children developed increased aggression or mania,[142] and there has been one report of psychotic deterioration in 2 children treated with buspirone for anxiety disorders.[143] Additional research on buspirone in children and adolescents would seem particularly worthwhile.

β-Blockers have been used with good effect for symptomatic relief in anxious younger patients with performance anxiety, hyperventilation syndrome and PTSD, as well as in an adolescent with multiple disabilities and self-injurious behaviour. However, they have been described as inhibiting TCA metabolism in 2 children who received propanolol 30 and 400 mg/day in combination with imipramine 75 and 80 mg/day, respectively.[144] Concentrations of imipramine were found to be near toxic in both cases. In addition, the risks of bradycardia, hypotension, bronchoconstriction in individuals with asthma, and neuroendocrine changes need to be borne in mind.[107]

Clonidine, an α_2-adrenergic agonist, has been used in the treatment of PTSD in younger patients. Concerns have been expressed about rebound hypertension following abrupt cessation of clonidine treatment, and electrocardiogram changes during treatment have been reported.[145] However, transient sedation appears to be the most commonly reported adverse effect when the medication is used in children with PTSD.[83] Overdose of clonidine can cause depressed level of consciousness, bradycardia, hypotension, transient hypertension, arrhythmia, respiratory depression, miosis and hypothermia.[146] Reports of sudden death due to acute cardiac failure in 4 children receiving a combination of clonidine and methylphenidate have stimulated intense and ongoing debate as to likely causality.[147]

MAOIs have also not been well studied in children and adolescents. While the difficulties of adhering to a strict diet make the irreversible MAOIs an unlikely choice except in the most refractory of cases, the introduction in some countries of a reversible inhibitor MAOI type A, with an apparently more favourable adverse effect profile, encourages research on the use of such agents in children and adolescents. Caution would have to be exercised with respect to sequential treatment with SSRIs, in view of the reported occurrence of the serotonin syndrome in such situations.[148]

Nefazodone, an antidepressant with both adrenergic and serotonergic effects, was found to be effective and well tolerated in a small case series of children and adolescents with social phobia.[49] The use of nefazodone[149,150] and venlafaxine[151] in depressed children and adolescents has been reported.

While antipsychotic drugs cannot be recommended for the treatment of anxiety disorders, they are often prescribed to young patients who have severe developmental disorders in which anxiety may be a prominent feature. The advent of novel antipsychotics, which appear to have a more benign adverse effect profile, would suggest that further research in this area is necessary. An open-label study in which 8 children, adolescents and adults who had pervasive developmental disorders were treated for 12 weeks with olanzepine (mean dosage 7.8 mg/day) found that anxiety symptoms, among others, were reduced by this medication. Adverse effects of increased appetite, weight gain and sedation were noted.[101]

3. Discussion

The usefulness of open trials and case reports is limited by several factors, including the possibility of spontaneous recovery from the conditions under consideration, noted to be 34% in the 1992 study by Keller et al.[2] However, even in the controlled trials which have been conducted, the number of participants is low, usually around 20, and very seldom more than 50 (table I). This seriously limits the statistical power of the studies, and thus their usefulness in establishing generalisable data concerning the outcome of anxiety disorders treated with pharmacotherapy in young patients.

On the basis of published controlled studies, the following can be inferred: clomipramine, fluoxetine and sertraline are effective in OCD; clonazepam is effective in the treatment of panic disorder; imipramine and possibly alprazolam are useful in school phobia, especially when there are comorbid anxiety disorders or depression; fluoxetine may be useful in selective mutism/social phobia; and clomipramine is effective in reducing stereotypies in autism.

As a starting point in management planning, it appears to be the consensus of clinicians treating children and adolescents with anxiety disorders that, should resources and symptom severity allow, psychotherapeutic treatment, usually cognitive-behavioural in nature, should be the initial intervention. Supportive and psycho-educational intervention with the family as well as the patient would appear to be mandatory whatever regimen is used.

If there is a need for more immediate relief of symptoms, or should psychotherapeutic treatment have failed to ameliorate the condition after an adequate trial, the addition of medication must be considered. Factors to be considered in the choice of medication should include age, safety data for that age-group, documented efficacy for the particular disorder in that age group, medical and psychiatric comorbidity, concurrent medication and the risk of drug-drug interactions,[152] inpatient or outpatient status, lethality in overdose, degree of supervision of medication if an outpatient, previous response to a particular type of medication and, all else being equal, financial implications.

Table I. Published controlled pharmacotherapy trials in anxiety disorders of childhood and adolescence

Year	Authors	Diagnosis	No. of pts	Medication(s) and dose (mean/range)	Duration (wks)	Outcome
1971	Gittelman-Klein & Klein[28]	School phobia	35	Imipramine 100-200mg vs placebo	6	Imipramine > placebo
1981	Berney et al.[30]	School phobia	46	Clomipramine 40-75mg vs placebo	12	No significant difference
1985	Flamentet al.[62]	OCD	19	Clomipramine 140mg vs placebo	10	Clomipramine > placebo
1989	Leonard et al.[63]	OCD	48	Clomipramine 150mg vs desipramine 155mg	10	Clomipramine > desipramine
1990	Bernstein et al.[34]	School refusal	24	Alprazolam 1-3mg vs imipramine 150-200mg vs placebo	8	Alprazolam > imipramine > placebo on clinician rating only
1992	Kutcher et al.[41]	Panic disorder	12	Clonazepam 1-2mg vs placebo	?	Clonazepam > placebo
1991	Leonard et al.[75]	OCD	26	Clomipramine 140mg vs imipramine 125mg	8 months	Clomipramine > imipramine
1992	De Veaugh-Geiss et al.[64]	OCD	60	Clomipramine 75-200mg vs placebo	8	Clomipramine > placebo
1992	Klein et al.[29]	Separation anxiety disorder	21	Imipramine 75-275mg vs placebo	6	No significant difference
1992	Kutcher et al.[41]	Panic disorder	12	Clonazepam 1-2mg vs placebo	?	Clonazepam > placebo
1992	Riddle et al.[65]	OCD	14	Fluoxetine 20mg vs placebo	20	Fluoxetine > placebo on CGI
1992	Simeon et al.[51]	Overanxious or avoidant disorder	30	Alprazolam 0.5-3.5mg vs placebo	4	No significant difference
1993	Gordon et al.[97]	Stereotypies in autistic disorder	12	Clomipramine 150mg vs placebo	10	Clomipramine > placebo
1993			12	Clomipramine 150mg vs desipramine 125mg	10	Clomipramine > imipramine
1993	Kurlan et al.[78]	OC symptoms in Tourette's	11	Fluoxetine 20-40mg vs placebo	4	No significant difference
1994	Black & Uhde[46]	Elective mutism	15	Fluoxetine 12-27mg vs placebo	12	Fluoxetine > placebo on parent ratings
1994	Graae et al.[33]	Separation anxiety	15	Clonazepam 0.5-2mg vs placebo	8	No significant difference
1996	Bouvard et al.[141]	Generalised anxiety disorder	42	Buspirone 30mg vs placebo	6	No significant difference
1998	March et al.[72]	OCD	187	Sertraline 25-200mg vs placebo	12	Sertraline > placebo
2000	Bernstein et al.[31]	School refusal + major depression and anxiety disorder	47	Imipramine + CBT vs placebo + CBT	8	Imipramine > placebo

CBT = cognitive behavioural therapy; CGI = Clinical Global Impression Scale; mo = months; OCD = obsessive-compulsive disorder; wks = weeks.

Treatment decisions are frequently made on the basis of the cost of individual drugs. However, in the longer term, multiple trials of cheaper but less effective medications may be just as costly as treatment with a more expensive but more effective, drug. Certainly, the high costs of many newer agents make the need for studies of efficacy and cost-efficiency paramount.

In children and adolescents with anxiety disorders, the immediate morbidity as well as the possible long term consequences of non-treatment need to be emphasised. Increasingly, these disorders are being shown to have significant impact on social and occupational functioning in some young patients. Furthermore, while there are relatively few long term follow-up studies of children and adolescents with anxiety disorders, a number of those published describe the persistence of original symptoms and the development of additional comorbid disorders.

Conversely, in considering pharmacotherapy of anxiety disorders in children and adolescents, several risks are apparent, some serious. In particular, the adverse cardiovascular effects of the TCAs and the risk of dependency with benzodiazepines have been stressed in the literature. The dearth of controlled clinical trials showing efficacy of medication over placebo also makes use of these agents problematic in many cases.

Predicting which drug is likely to be the most effective for a particular child is not currently possible. The drugs discussed above act on different neurotransmitter systems: adrenergic, serotonergic and γ-aminobutyric acid (GABA)-ergic, and may thus have their effects at different levels of symptom production. Detailed elaboration of the mechanism of action, safety and efficacy of drugs in children and adolescents, as well as further rigorous controlled studies of pharmacotherapy alone and together with psychotherapy, is necessary before evidence-based decisions can be made in clinical practice.

Acknowledgements

Dr Stein is supported by a grant from the Medical Research Council Research Unit on Anxiety and Stress Disorders (South Africa).

References

1. Myers JK, Weissman MM, Tischler GL, et al. Six month prevalence of psychiatric disorders in three communities. Arch Gen Psychiatry 1984; 41: 959-67
2. Keller MB, Lavori PW, Wunder J, et al. Chronic course of anxiety disorders in children and adolescents. J Am Acad Child Adolesc Psychiatry 1992; 31: 595-9
3. McGee R, Feehan M, Williams S, et al. DSM III disorders in a large sample of adolescents. J Am Acad Child Adolesc Psychiatry 1990; 29: 611-9
4. Kearney CA, Silverman WK. A critical review of pharmacotherapy for youth with anxiety disorders: things are not as they seem. J Anxiety Disord 1998; 12: 83-102
5. Kendall PC, Flannery-Schroeder EC. Methodological issues in treatment research for anxiety disorders in youth. J Abnorm Child Psychol 1998; 26: 27-38
6. Greenhill LL, Pine D, March J, et al. Assessment issues in treatment research of pediatric anxiety disorders: what is working, what is not working, what is missing and what needs improvement. Psychopharmacol Bull 1998; 34: 155-64
7. Allen AJ, Leonard H, Swedo SE. Current knowledge of medications for the treatment of childhood anxiety disorders. J Am Acad Child Adolesc Psychiatry 1995; 34: 976-86
8. Arnold LE, Stoff DM, Cook E, et al. Ethical issues in biological psychiatric research with children and adolescents. J Am Acad Child Adolesc Psychiatry 1995; 34: 929-39
9. Kashani JH, Orvaschel H. A community study of anxiety in children and adolescents. Am J Psychiatry 1990; 147: 313-8
10. Weissman MM, Wickramaratne P, Warner V, et al. Assessing psychiatric disorders in children. Arch Gen Psychiatry 1987; 4: 747-53
11. American Psychiatric Association. Diagnostic and statistical manual of mental disorders. 3rd ed. Washington, DC: American Psychiatric Association, 1980
12. Simonoff E, Pickles A, Meyer JM, et al. The Virginia twin study of adolescent behavioral development. Arch Gen Psychiatry 1997; 54: 801-8
13. Mattison RE. Suicide and other consequences of childhood and adolescent anxiety disorders. J Clin Psychiatry 1988; 49: 9-11
14. Last CG, Hansen C, Franco N. Anxious children in adulthood: a prospective study of adjustment. J Am Acad Child Adolesc Psychiatry 1997; 36: 645-52
15. Kasen S, Cohen P, Skodol AE, et al. Influence of child and adolescent psychiatric disorders on young adult personality disorder. Am J Psychiatry 1999; 156: 1529-35
16. American Psychiatric Association. Diagnostic and statistical manual of mental disorders. 3rd rev. ed. Washington, DC: American Psychiatric Association, 1987
17. American Psychiatric Association. Diagnostic and statistical manual of mental disorders. 4th ed. Washington, DC: American Psychiatric Association, 1994
18. Kendall PC. Treating anxiety disorders in children: results of a randomized clinical trial. J Consult Clin Psychol 1994; 62: 100-10
19. Kendall PC, Flannery-Schroeder E, Panichelli-Mindel SM, et al. Therapy for youths with anxiety disorders: a second randomized clinical trial. J Consult Clin Psychol 1997; 65: 366-80
20. Silverman WK, Kurtines WM, Ginsburg GS et al. Treating anxiety disorders in children with group cognitive-behavioural therapy: a randomized clinical trial. J Consult Clin Psychol 1999; 67: 995-1003
21. March JS, Amaya-Jackson L, Murray MC, et al. Cognitive-behavioral psychotherapy for children and adolescents with posttraumatic stress disorder after a single incident stressor. J Am Acad Child Adolesc Psychiatry 1998; 37: 585-93
22. Target M, Fonagy P. Efficacy of psychoanalysis for children with emotional disorders. J Am Acad Child Adolesc Psychiatry 1994; 33: 361-71
23. Mitchell J, McCauley E, Burke PM, et al. Phenomenology of depression in children and adolescents. J Am Acad Child Adolesc Psychiatry 1988; 27: 12-20
24. Gittelman R, Klein DF. Relationship between separation anxiety and panic and agoraphobic disorders. Psychopathology 1984; 17 Suppl.: 56-65
25. Weissman MM, Leckman JF, Merikangas KR, et al. Depression and anxiety disorders in parents and children. Arch Gen Psychiatry 1984; 41: 845-52
26. Kraft I. A clinical study of chlordiazepoxide used in psychiatric disorders of children. Int J Neuropsychiatry 1965; 1: 433-7
27. D'Amato G. Chlordiazepoxide in management of school phobia. Dis Nerv Sys 1962; 23: 292-5
28. Gittelman-Klein R, Klein DF. Controlled imipramine treatment of school phobia. Arch Gen Psychiatry 1971; 25: 204-7
29. Klein RG, Koplewicz HS, Kanner A. Imipramine treatment of children with separation anxiety disorder. J Am Acad Child Adolesc Psychiatry 1992; 31: 21-8
30. Berney T, Kolvin I, Bhate SR, et al. School phobia: a therapeutic trial with clomipramine and short term outcome. Br J Psychiatry 1981; 138: 110-8
31. Bernstein GA, Borchardt CM, Perwien AR, et al. Imipramine plus cognitive-behavioral therapy in the treatment of school refusal. J Am Acad Child Adolesc Psychiatry 2000; 39: 276-83
32. Biederman J. Clonazepam in the treatment of prepubertal children with panic-like symptoms. J Clin Psychiatry 1987; 48 Suppl.: 38-42

33. Graae F, Milner J, Rizzotto L, et al. Clonazepam in childhood anxiety disorders. J Am Acad Child Adolesc Psychiatry 1994; 33: 372-6
34. Bernstein GA, Garfinkel BD, Borchardt CM. Comparative studies of pharmacotherapy for school refusal. J Am Acad Child Adolesc Psychiatry 1990; 29: 773-81
35. Birmaher B, Waterman GS, Ryan N, et al. Fluoxetine for childhood anxiety disorders. J Am Acad Child Adolesc Psychiatry 1994; 33: 993-9
36. Fairbanks JM, Pine DS, Tancer NK, et al. Open fluoxetine treatment of mixed anxiety disorders in children and adolescents. J Child Adolesc Psychopharmacol 1997; 7: 17-29
37. Black B, Robbins DR. Panic disorder in children and adolescents. J Am Acad Child Adolesc Psychiatry 1990; 29: 36-44
38. Garland EJ, Smith DH. Case Study: panic disorder on a child psychiatry consultation service. J Am Acad Child Adolesc Psychiatry 1990; 29: 785-8
39. Ballenger JC, Carek DJ, Steele JJ, et al. Three cases of panic disorder with agoraphobia in children. Am J Psychiatry 1989; 146: 922-4
40. Kutcher SP, Mackenzie S. Successful clonazepam treatment of adolescents with panic disorder. J Clin Psychopharmacol 1988; 8: 299-301
41. Kutcher SP, Reiter S, Gardner DM, et al. The pharmacotherapy of anxiety disorders in children and adolescents. Psychiatr Clin North Am 1992; 15: 41-67
42. Joorabchi B. Expressions of the hyperventilation syndrome in childhood. Clin Paediatr 1977; 16: 1110-5
43. Gorman JM. The use of newer antidepressants for panic disorder. J Clin Psychiatry 1997; 58 Suppl. 14: 54-8
44. Black B, Uhde TW. Case study: elective mutism as a variant of social phobia. J Am Acad Child Adolesc Psychiatry 1992; 31: 1090-4
45. Dummit ES, Klein RG, Tancer NK, et al. Fluoxetine treatment of children with selective mutism: an open trial. J Am Acad Child Adolesc Psychiatry 1996; 35: 615-21
46. Black B, Uhde TW. Treatment of elective mutism with fluoxetine: a double-blind, placebo-controlled study. J Am Acad Child Adolesc Psychiatry 1994; 33: 1000-6
47. Campbell M, Cueva JE. Psychopharmacology in child and adolescent psychiatry: a review of the past seven years. Pt II. J Am Acad Child Adolesc Psychiatry 1995; 34: 1262-72
48. Lafferty JE, Constantino JN. Fluvoxamine in selective mutism [letter]. J Am Acad Child Adolesc Psychiatry 1998; 37: 12-3
49. Mancini C, Van Ameringen M, Oakman JM, et al. Serotonergic agents in the treatment of social phobia in children and adolescents: a case series. Depress Anxiety 1999; 10: 33-9
50. Zwier KJ, Rao U. Buspirone use in an adolescent with social phobia and mixed personality disorder (cluster A type). J Am Acad Child Adolesc Psychiatry 1994; 33: 1007-11
51. Simeon JG, Ferguson HB, Knott V, et al. Clinical, cognitive and neurophysiological effects of alprazolam in children and adolescents with overanxious and avoidant disorders. J Am Acad Child Adolesc Psychiatry 1992; 31: 29-33
52. Liebowitz MR, Schneier F, Campeas R, et al. Phenelzine vs atenolol in social phobia: a placebo-controlled comparison. Arch Gen Psychiatry 1992; 49: 290-300
53. Golwyn DH, Weinstock RC. Phenelzine treatment of elective mutism: a case report. J Clin Psychiatry 1990; 51: 384-5
54. Rupp SN. Haloperidol for Tourette's disorder plus selective mutism. J Am Acad Child Adolesc Psychiatry 1999; 38: 7
55. Noyes Jr R. Beta-adrenergic blockers. In: Last CG, Hersen M, editors. Handbook of anxiety disorders. New York: Pergamon Press, 1988: 445-59
56. Krishan G. Oxprenolol in the treatment of examination stress. Curr Med Res Opin 1976; 4: 241-3
57. Black B, Uhde TW, Tancer ME. Fluoxetine for the treatment of social phobia. J Clin Psychopharmacol 1992; 12: 293-5
58. Baldwin D, Bobes J, Stein DJ, et al. Paroxetine in social phobia/social anxiety disorder: randomised, double-blind, placebo-controlled study. Br J Psychiatry 1999; 175: 120-6
59. Bernstein G, Shaw KS. American Academy of Child and Adolescent Psychiatry: practice parameters for the assessment and treatment of anxiety disorders. J Am Acad Child Adolesc Psychiatry 1993; 32: 1089-97
60. Balon R. Fluvoxamine for phobia of storms. Acta Psychiatr Scand 1999; 100: 244-5
61. Avci A, Diler RS, Tamam L. Fluoxetine treatment in a 2.5-year-old girl. J Am Acad Child Adolesc Psychiatry 1998; 37: 901-2
62. Flament MF, Rapoport JL, Berg CJ, et al. Clomipramine treatment of childhood obsessive-compulsive disorder: a double-blind controlled study. Arch Gen Psychiatry 1985; 42: 977-83
63. Leonard HL, Swedo SE, Rapoport JL, et al. Treatment of obsessive-compulsive disorder with clomipramine and desipramine in children and adolescents: a double-blind crossover comparison. Arch Gen Psychiatry 1989; 46: 1088-92
64. De Veaugh-Geiss J, Moroz G, Biederman J, et al. Clomipramine hydrochloride in childhood and adolescent obsessive-compulsive disorder: a multi-centre trial. J Am Acad Child Adolesc Psychiatry 1992; 31: 45-9
65. Riddle MA, Scahill L, King RA, et al. Double-blind, crossover trial of fluoxetine and placebo in children and adolescents with obsessive-compulsive disorder. J Am Acad Child Adolesc Psychiatry 1992; 31: 1062-9
66. Geller DA, Biederman J, Reed ED, et al. Similarities in response to fluoxetine in the treatment of children and adolescents with obsessive-compulsive disorder. J Am Acad Child Adolesc Psychiatry 1995; 34: 36-44
67. Apter A, Ratzoni G, King RA, et al. Fluvoxamine open-label treatment of adolescent inpatients with obsessive-compulsive disorder or depression. J Am Acad Child Adolesc Psychiatry 1994; 33: 342-8
68. Alderman J, Wolkow R, Johnston H, et al. Sertraline treatment in children and adolescents: tolerability, efficacy and pharmacokinetics. Eur Neuropsychopharmacol 1996; 6 Suppl. 3: 11-2
69. Thomsen PH. Child and adolescent obsessive-compulsive disorder treated with citalopram: findings from an open trial of 23 cases. J Child Adolesc Psychopharmacol 1997; 7: 157-66
70. Riddle MA, Claghorn J, Gaffney G, et al. Fluvoxamine for children and adolescents with obsessive-compulsive disorder: a controlled multi-center trial. Scientific Proceedings of the 1996 Annual Meeting of the American Academy of Child and Adolescent Psychiatry XII, 110-11
71. Wolkow R, March J, Biederman J. A placebo-controlled trial of sertraline treatment for pediatric obsessive-compulsive disorder. Abstracted in the 6th World Congress of Biological Psychiatry, Nice, France; 1997; 42: 213S
72. March JS, Biederman J, Wolkow R, et al. Sertraline in children and adolescents with obsessive-compulsive disorder: a multicenter randomized controlled trial. JAMA 1998; 280: 1752-6
73. Rosenberg DR, Stewart CM, Fitzgerald KD, et al. Paroxetine open-label treatment of pediatric outpatients with obsessive-compulsive disorder. J Am Acad Child Adolesc Psychiatry 1999; 38: 118-5

74. Figueroa Y, Rosenberg DR, Birmaher B, et al. Combination treatment with clomipramine and selective serotonin reuptake inhibitors for obsessive-compulsive disorder in children and adolescents. J Child Adolesc Psychopharmacol 1998; 8: 61-7
75. Leonard HL, Swedo SE, Lenane MC, et al. A double-blind desipramine substitution during long-term clomipramine treatment in children and adolescents with obsessive compulsive disorder. Arch Gen Psychiatry 1991; 48: 922-7
76. March JS. Cognitive-behavioural psychotherapy for children and adolescents with OCD: a review and recommendations for treatment. J Am Acad Child Adolesc Psychiatry 1995; 34: 7-18
77. McDougle CJ, Goodman WK, Leckman JF, et al. Haloperidol addition in fluvoxamine-refractory obsessive-compulsive disorder: a double-blind placebo-controlled study in patients with and without tics. Arch Gen Psychiatry 1994; 51: 302-8
78. Kurlan R, Como PG, Deeley C, et al. A pilot controlled study of fluoxetine for obsessive-compulsive symptoms in children with Tourette's syndrome. Clin Neuropharmacol 1993; 16: 167-72
79. Eapen V, Trimble MR, Robertson MM. The use of fluoxetine in Gilles de la Tourette syndrome and obsessive compulsive behaviours: preliminary clinical experience. Prog Neurpsychopharmacol Biol Psychiatry 1996; 20: 737-43
80. Hawkridge S, Stein DJ, Bouwer C. Combined pharmacotherapy for TS and OCD [letter]. J Am Acad Child Adolesc Psychiatry 1996; 35: 703-4
81. Leonard HL. New developments in the treatment of obsessive-compulsive disorder. J Clin Psychiatry 1997; 58 Suppl. 14: 39-45
82. Famularo R, Kinscherff R, Fenton T. Propanolol treatment for childhood posttraumatic stress disorder, acute type: a pilot study. Am J Dis Chil 1988; 142: 1244-7
83. Harmon RJ, Riggs PD. Clonidine for posttraumatic stress disorder in preschool children. J Am Acad Child Adolesc Psychiatry 1996; 35: 1247-9
84. Donnelly CL, Amaya-Jackson L, March JS. Psychopharmacology of pediatric posttraumatic stress disorder. J Child Adolesc Psychopharmacol 1999; 9: 203-20
85. Marshall RD, Stein DJ, Liebowitz MR, et al. Psychopharmacology of posttraumatic stress disorder. Psychiatric Annals 1996; 26: 217-26
85a. Seedat S, Lockhart R, Kaminer D, et al. An open trial of citalopram in adolescents with posttraumatic stress disorder. Int Clin Psychopharmacol. In press
86. Simeon JG, Ferguson HB. Alprazolam effects in children with anxiety disorders. Can J Psychiatry 1987; 32: 570-4
87. Lader M, Scotto JC. A multicentre double-blinded comparison of hydroxyzine, busprione and placebo in patients with generalized anxiety disorder. Psychopharmacology Berl 1998; 139: 402-6
88. Kranzler H. Use of buspirone in an adolescent with overanxious disorder. J Am Acad Child Adolesc Psychiatry 1988; 27: 789-90
89. Hanna GL, Fluent TE, Fischer DJ. Separation anxiety in children and adolescents treated with risperidone. J Child Adolesc Psychopharmacol 1999; 9: 277-83
90. Hanna GL, Feibusch EL, Albright KJ. Buspirone treatment of anxiety associated with pharyngeal dysphagia in a four-year-old. J Child Adolesc Psychopharmacol 1997; 7: 137-43
91. Cook EH, Rowlet R, Jaselskis C, et al. Fluoxetine treatment of children and adults with autistic disorder and mental retardation. J Am Acad Child Adolesc Psychiatry 1992; 31: 739-45
92. Dech B, Budow L. The use of fluoxetine in an adolescent with Prader-Willi Syndrome. J Am Acad Child Adolesc Psychiatry 1991; 30: 298-302
93. Garber HJ, McGonigle JJ, Slomka GT, et al. Clomipramine treatment of stereotypic behaviours and self-injury in patients with developmental disabilities. J Am Acad Child Adolesc Psychiatry 1992; 31: 1157-60
94. Steingard RJ, Zimitsky B, DeMaso D, et al. Sertraline treatment of transition-associated anxiety and agitation in children with autistic disorder. J Child Adolesc Psychopharmacology 1997; 7: 9-15
95. Mehlinger R, Scheftner WA, Poznanski E. Fluoxetine and autism [letter]. J Am Acad Child Adolesc Psychiatry 1990; 29: 985
96. Todd RD. Fluoxetine in autism [letter]. Am J Psychiatry 1991; 148: 1089
97. Gordon CT, State RC, Nelson JE, et al. A double-blind comparison of clomipramine, desipramine and placebo in the treatment of autistic disorder. Arch Gen Psychiatry 1993; 50: 441-7
98. McDougle CJ, Naylor ST, Cohen DJ, et al. A double-blind, placebo-controlled study of fluvoxamine in adults with autistic disorder. Arch Gen Psychiatry 1996; 53: 1001-8
99. Lang C, Remington D. Treatment with propanolol of severe self-injurious behaviour in a blind, deaf, retarded adolescent. J Am Acad Child Adolesc Psychiatry 1994; 33: 265-9
100. Szabo CP, Bracken C. Imipramine and Asperger's [letter]. J Am Acad Child Adolesc Psychiatry 1994; 33: 431-2
101. Potenza MN, Holmes JP, Kanes SJ, et al. Olanzapine treatment of children, adolescents and adults with pervasive developmental disorders: an open-label pilot study. J Clin Psychopharmacol 1999; 19: 37-44
102. Lucas AR, Pasley FC. Psychoactive drugs in the treatment of emotionally disturbed children: haloperidol and diazepam. Compr Psychiatry 1969; 10: 376-86
103. Commander M, Green SH, Prendergast M. Behavioural disturbances in children treated with clonazepam. Dev Med Child Neurol 1991; 33: 362-3
104. Reiter S, Kutcher S. Disinhibition and anger outbursts in adolescents treated with clonazepam. J Clin Psychopharmacol 1991; 11: 268
105. Pfefferbaum B, Butler PM, Mullins D, et al. Two cases of benzodiazepine toxicity in children. J Clin Psychiatry 1987; 48: 450-2
106. Lechin F, van der Bijs B, Benaim M. Benzodiazepines: tolerability in elderly patients. Psychother Psychosom 1996; 65: 171-82
107. Riddle MA, Bernstein GA, Cook EH, et al. Anxiolytics, adrenergic agents and naltrexone. J Am Acad Child Adolesc Psychiatry 1999; 38: 546-56
108. Cruz R. Clomipramine side effects [letter]. J Am Acad Child Adolesc Psychiatry 1992; 31: 1168-9
109. Alarcon RD, Johnson BR, Lucas JP. Paranoid and aggressive behavior in two obsessive/compulsive adolescents treated with clomipramine. J Am Acad Child Adolesc Psychiatry 1991; 30: 999-1002
110. Tingelstad JB. The cardiotoxicity of the tricyclics. J Am Acad Child Adolesc Psychiatry 1991; 30: 845-6
111. Biederman J, Gastfriend D, Jellinek MS, et al. Cardiovascular effects of desipramine in children and adolescents with attention deficit disorder. J Pediatr 1985; 106: 1017-20
112. Preskorn SH, Weller EB, Weller RA, et al. Plasma levels of imipramine and adverse effects in children. Am J Psychiatry 1983; 140: 1332-5
113. Walsh BT, Greenhill LL, Giardina EGV, et al. Effects of desipramine on autonomic input to the heart. J Am Acad Child Adolesc Psychiatry 1999; 38: 1186-92
114. Mezzacappa E, Steingard R, Kindlon D, et al. Tricyclic antidepressants and cardiac autonomic control in children and adolescents. J Am Acad Child Adolesc Psychiatry 1998; 37: 52-9

115. Waslick BD, Walsh BT, Greenhill LL, et al. Cardiovascular effects of desipramine in children and adults during exercise testing. J Am Acad Child Adolesc Psychiatry 1999; 38: 179-86
116. Bartels MG, Varley CK, Mitchell J, et al. Pediatric cardiovascular effects of imipramine and desipramine. J Am Acad Child Adolesc Psychiatry 1991; 30: 100-3
117. Wamboldt MZ, Yancey Jr AG, Roesler TA. Cardiovascular effects of tricyclic antidepressants in childhood asthma: a case series and review. J Child Adolesc Psychopharmacol 1997; 7: 45-64
118. Riddle MA, Nelson JC, Kleinman CS, et al. Sudden death in children receiving Norpramin®: a review of three reported cases and commentary. J Am Acad Child Adolesc Psychiatry 1991; 30: 104-8
119. Biederman J, Thisted RA, Greenhill LL, et al. Estimation of the association between desipramine and the risk for sudden death in 5- to 14-year old children. J Clin Psychiatry 1995; 56: 87-93
120. Leonard HL, Meyer MC, Swedo SE, et al. Electrocardiographic changes during desipramine and clomipramine treatment in children and adolescents. J Am Acad Child Adolesc Psychiatry 1995; 34: 1460-8
121. Cohen LG, Biederman J, Wilens TE, et al. Desipramine clearance in children and adolescents: absence of effect of development and gender. J Am Acad Child Adolesc Psychiatry 1999; 38: 79-85
122. Riddle M, King RA, Hardin MT, et al. Behavioral side effects of fluoxetine in children and adolescents. J Child Adolesc Psychopharmacology 1991; 1: 193-8
123. King RA, Riddle MA, Chappell PB, et al. Emergence of self-destructive phenomena in children and adolescents during fluoxetine treatment. J Am Acad Child Adolesc Psychiatry 1991; 30: 179-86
124. Walkup JT. A differential diagnosis of the adverse behavioural effects of fluoxetine. Newsl Am Acad Child Adolesc Psychiatry 1994; 25: 28-30
125. Constantino JN, Liberman M, Kincaid M. Effects of serotonin reuptake inhibitors on aggressive behaviour in psychiatrically hospitalized adolescents: results of an open trial. J Child Adolesc Psychopharmacol 1997; 7: 31-44
126. Ambrosini PJ, Wagner KD, Biederman J, et al. Multicentre open-label sertraline study in adolescent outpatients with major depression. J Am Acad Child Adolesc Psychiatry 1999; 38: 566-72
127. Heimann SW, March JS. SSRI-induced mania [letter]. J Am Acad Child Adolesc Psychiatry 1996; 35: 4
128. Diler RS, Avci A. SSRI-induced mania in obsessive-compulsive disorder [letter]. J Amer Acad Child Adolesc Psychiatry 1999; 38: 6-7
129. Leo RJ. Movement disorders associated with the serotonin selective reuptake inhibitors. J Clin Psychiatry 1996; 57: 449-54
130. Bates GDL, Khin-Maung-Zaw F. Movement disorder with fluoxetine. J Am Acad Child Adolesc Psychiatry 1998; 37: 14-5
131. Rey-Sanchez F, Gutierrez-Casares JR. Paroxetine in children with major depressive disorder: an open trial. J Am Acad Child Adolesc Psychiatry 1997; 36: 1443-7
132. Jain U, Birmaher B, Garcia M, et al. Fluoxetine: a chart review of efficacy and adverse effects. J Child Adolesc Psychopharmacology 1993; 2: 259-65
133. Gitlin MJ. Psychotropic medications and their effects on sexual function: diagnosis, biology, and treatment approaches. J Clin Psychiatry 1995; 56: 536-7
134. Carek DJ. SSRI and sexual functioning. J Am Acad Child Adolesc Psychiatry 1996; 35: 1106-7
135. Bangs ME, Petti TA, Janus M-D. Fluoxetine-induced memory impairment in an adolescent. J Am Acad Child Adolesc Psychiatry 1994; 33: 1303-6
136. Campbell-Carol NB, Franco KN, Tamburrino MB, et al. Vital signs on antidepressants [letter]. J Am Acad Child Adolesc Psychiatry 1998; 37: 13-4
137. Wilens TE, Biederman J, March JS, et al. Absence of cardiovascular adverse effects of sertraline in children and adolescents. J Am Acad Child Adolesc Psychiatry 1999; 38: 573-7
138. Gracious BL. Atrioventricular nodal re-entrant tachycardia associated with stimulant treatment. J Child Adolesc Psychopharmacol 1999; 9: 125-8
139. Myers LB, Krenzelok EP. Paroxetine (Paxil) overdose: a pediatric focus. Vet Hum Toxicol 1997; 39: 86-8
140. Haddad P. Newer antidepressants and the discontinuation syndrome. J Clin Psychiatry 1997; 58 Suppl. 7: 17-21
141. Bouvard MP, Braconnier A-J, Dissoubray C. Buspirone in adolescents with anxiety disorders [abstract]. American Psychiatric Association 149th Annual Meeting, New York: 1996, May 4-9: AP4
142. Pfeffer CR, Jiang H, Domeshek LJ. Buspirone treatment of psychiatrically hospitalized prepubertal children with symptoms of anxiety and aggression. J Child Adolesc Psychopharmacol 1997; 7: 145-55
143. Soni P, Weintraub AL. Buspirone-associated mental status changes. J Am Acad Child Adolesc Psychiatry 1992; 31: 1098-9
144. Gillette DW, Tannery LP. Beta blocker inhibits tricyclic metabolism. J Am Acad Child Adolesc Psychiatry 1994; 33: 223-4
145. Chandron KSK. ECG and clonidine. J Am Acad Child Adolesc Psychiatry 1994; 33: 1351-2
146. Nichols MH, King WD, James LP. Clonidine poisoning in Jefferson County, Alabama. Ann Emerg Med 1997; 29: 511-7
147. Wilens TE, Spencer TJ, Swanson JM, et al. Combining methyl phenidate and clonidine (debate forum). J Am Acad Child Adolesc Psychiatry 1999; 38: 614-22
148. Sternbach H. The serotonin syndrome. Am J Psychiatry 1991; 148: 705-13
149. Wilens TE, Spencer TJ, Biederman J, et al. Case study: nefazodone for juvenile mood disorders. J Am Acad Child Adolesc Psychiatry 1997; 36: 481-5
150. Findling RL, Magnus RD, Preskorn SH, et al. Open pharmacokinetic study of nefazodone in children and adolescents with depression [abstract NR-96]. American Academy of Child and Adolescent Psychiatry 44th Annual Meeting, Toronto: 1997, October
151. Mandoki MW, Tapia MR, Tapia MA, et al. Venlafaxine in the treatment of children and adolescents with major depression. Psychopharmacol Bull 1997; 33: 149-54
152. Ten Eick AP, Nakamura H, Reed MD. Drug-drug interactions in paediatric psychopharmacology. Pediatr Clin North Am 1998; 45: 1233-64

Correspondence: Dr *Susan M. Hawkridge*, Department of Psychiatry, University of Stellenbosch, PO Box 19063, Tygerberg 7505, South Africa.
E-mail: smh@gerga.sun.ac.za

Bipolar Disorder in Children and Adolescents
A Guide to Diagnosis and Treatment

Raul R. Silva, Fredrick Matzner, Jose Diaz, Sanjay Singh and
E. Steven Dummit III

New York University School of Medicine, Division of Child and Adolescent Psychiatry,
New York, New York, USA

1. Diagnosis

Historically, there have been case reports of mania in children as far back as the late nineteenth century,[1] although whether such reports would match our current conceptualisation of mania as a distinct mood disorder has not been established. Descriptions of mental illness linking mania and melancholia in adults have been traced in the literature back to the Hippocratic writers of ancient Greece. However, the distinction between such 'circular' types of illness and the chronic deteriorating course of 'dementia praecox', or schizophrenia, awaited the seminal description of manic-depressive illness by Emil Kraepelin at the dawn of the twentieth century.[2] Prior to this, 'mania' was typically used as a general term for mad, rageful, intoxicated or excited behavioural dyscontrol and was not exclusively linked to elated or an expansive change in mood as a specific psychiatric syndrome.[3]

While the adolescent onset of manic-depressive disorder was common in the 900 cases reported by Kraepelin in 1921, cases with onset prior to age 10 years were rare, at 0.4%.[2] Recently, increasing numbers of cases of bipolar disorder have been reported in children younger than 10 years.[4,5] These reports have sparked controversy, in part due to their inconsistency with epidemiological and longitudinal studies and the historic rarity of clear prepubertal cases of mania described in the literature. While childhood depression was also once thought to be rare, systematic research in recent years has established the validity of unipolar mood disorders in prepubertal children.[6] Similar systematic and methodologically rigorous research into bipolar affective disorders of childhood is less common.

A comprehensive review of reports pertaining to bipolar disorder in children and adolescents is beyond the scope of this paper, and the reader is referred to several thorough recent reviews for such detail.[7-10] We instead examine the controversy surrounding prepubertal mania and describe the view of childhood bipolar disorder that is emerging from the scientific literature.

1.1 Assessment and Diagnosis

According to DSM-IV,[11] the diagnostic criteria for mania in children differ little from those in adults. Mania is manifested by:

- a distinct period of abnormally and persistently elevated, expansive or irritable mood, lasting at least 1 week (or any duration if hospitalisation is necessary) [A criterion]
- accompanied by three (or four if mood is only irritable) of the following symptoms (B criterion): inflated self-esteem and grandiosity, decrease need for sleep, increased talkativeness or pressure to keep talking, racing thoughts or flight of ideas, distractibility, increased goal-directed activity or psychomotor agitation, and excessive involvement in pleasurable activity with high potential for painful consequences.

The mood disturbance must be sufficiently severe to cause marked psychosocial or occupational impairment, or be accompanied by psychotic symptoms or result in hospitalisation.

Excluded from the diagnosis are individuals with symptoms due to the direct physiological effects of substance use, medication or medical conditions such as endocrine or neurological disorders. Patients with psychosocial impairment and less than full criteria for mania are considered hypomanic. The absence of full manic episodes in the presence of hypomania alternating with full major depressive episodes is labelled 'bipolar type II', while chronic symptoms of cycling between hypomania and dysthymic mild states of depression is labelled 'cyclothymia'. The significance of these distinctions in childhood has not been studied.

DSM-IV also provides a category for 'mixed episode', which represents the concurrent presence of symptoms meeting criteria for both manic episode and major depressive episode for at least a week, although fewer empirical studies have been published about this diagnostic category and the clinical utility of a separate category is not well defined.[12,13]

Many authors have reported that mixed states of irritability and manic behaviour with tantrums, affective storminess, and defiant or aggressive behaviour problems are more common in childhood and may account for the failure of clinicians to recognise mania in children with disruptive behaviour.[7,10,12]

Rapid cycling, where many manic episodes per year occur, or switching between manic and depressed phases occurs constantly, is also reported in children and adolescents.[7] Mixed presentations and rapid cycling in adolescents may increase the risk of relapse. Akiskal[14] has theorised that childhood-onset depression, rapid cycling and mixed features signify a more virulent familial form of cyclic affective disorder, which is associated with 'hyperthymic temperament' that leads to externalising behaviour, in contrast with anxious, phobic, internalising psychopathology which is more common in unipolar pedigrees. This confluence of mood and externalising behavioural features lies at the heart of the current debate about prepubertal mania.

1.1.1 Juvenile Mania – Diagnostic Controversy

The difficulty in diagnosing mania in children has been noted in nonsystematic case reports for several decades.[10] In recent years some researchers have suggested that many young children with mania may be mistakenly diagnosed with attention deficit hyperactivity disorder (ADHD).[4,5] This view has arisen because of the overlap of diagnostic criteria and symptoms of the two disorders. Children with ADHD typically have distractibility, talkativeness, decreased and restless sleep, very high motor activity, and impulsive pleasure-seeking behaviour which results in negative social consequences. Frequently, the consequences of their behaviour and academic difficulties lead to angry interactions with others and cause dysphoria in the hyperactive child. ADHD is a chronic disorder, in which the core symptoms are not episodic in nature, although associated anger and irritability could appear to be episodic if related to the social and environmental consequences.

Because of the high rates of endorsement of irritability and the B criteria for mania in structured interviews of parents and children referred for hyperactivity, aggressivity and disruptive behaviour, Biederman et al.[15] have begun to refer to this constellation of hyperactivity and irritability as 'juvenile mania'. These investigators have suggested that the rarity of mania in children could be due to clinician bias against the diagnosis and in favour of 'bad ADHD' as an explanation of the severity of such cases.[16]

The current controversy over the diagnosis of juvenile mania centres on two issues. The first issue is the quality of affective symptoms, namely euphoric or elated mood versus irritability and chronic anger. The second issue is the temporal course of the affective symptoms, whether they occur as distinct acute episodes or are chronically present. Supporters of the juvenile mania diagnosis[7,15] argue that mania can be diagnosed in chronically hyperactive and irritable children who meet criteria for ADHD, without the presence of a cyclic course of euphoria and depression and the distinct episodic changes in affect and behaviour that typify the presentation in adults. Evidence for this view includes: (i) the high rates of comorbidity of ADHD and mania reported in structured interviews of children and adolescents clinically referred for either ADHD or bipolar disorder;[5,17,18] (ii) higher rates of both disorders in families of children with ADHD and bipolar compared with those in controls;[19] (iii) a retrospective report of higher rates of childhood hyperactivity symptoms in adults with bipolar compared with unipolar disorder;[20] and (iv) anecdotal reports of response of such children to antimanic treatments, such as lithium.

The arguments against viewing this presentation of irritability and hyperactivity as a variant of mania are both nosological and empirical. If the A criterion requiring a distinct period of changed affect is discarded, then the phenomenology of such cases cannot be equivalent to the validated syndrome of bipolar manic illness in adults. Indeed, such cases could not be viewed as having a bipolar course of illness if affect does not undergo cyclic change. Such a conceptualisation would discard the fundamental nosological advance made by Kraepelin[2] when he distinguished manic depression from chronic schizophrenic and organic forms of psychotic illness. This would represent a step backward to the era when 'mania' referred to any extreme behavioural disturbance.[3] Mania categorically has not been viewed as a stable state, and it seems unwise to do so now without substantial evidence that such patients progress to have more typical bipolar courses in adolescence or adulthood.[16]

Many retrospective studies of adults with bipolar disorder have examined the issue of age of onset[2] and have consistently found extremely low numbers who report onset before the age of 10 years, in the range below 1% as originally documented by Kraepelin.[2] No epidemiological study of children has found prepubertal mania, despite using structured interview methodologies similar to the clinical data from Biederman's group.[16] This weighs against the possibility that juvenile mania is misdiagnosed in clinical settings because of clinician bias.

Finally, a substantial literature on the use of lithium for aggressive behaviour in children existed before the current debate about juvenile mania.[21,22] None of the researchers involved in lithium trials with children ever suggested that what they were treating was mania or that lithium is specifically efficacious only for bipolar disorder.[23]

The issue of using the diagnosis of mania in hyperactive children is not trivial. Besides the importance of refining a scientific nosology in our field, it is also important to consider the ramifications of the diagnostic label given to a patient. The utility of psychostimulants for hyperactive and disruptive behaviours in childhood has been known for longer than any other modern psychotropic medication, having first been reported in 1937.[24] Hundreds of studies of psychostimulants have documented the efficacy and safety of these agents in children. The commonly used mood-stabilising medications for bipolar disorder (lithium, anticonvulsants and antipsychotics) can have unpleasant and dangerous short and long term adverse effects (see section 3.2), as well as being lethal in overdosage. Furthermore, comparatively few scientific studies have demonstrated the safety and efficacy of these medications in childhood disorders. It would be imprudent to expose a child to these risks without being certain that disordered behaviour is due to affective dysregulation rather than the much more common syndrome of chronic hyperactivity.

Although bipolar disorder and ADHD are both usually chronic disorders, the prognosis and risk of comorbid disorders both differ in childhood and later in adulthood. Besides pharmacological management, the two disorders may require different psychosocial interventions to optimise outcome. For a more thorough discussion of this diagnostic controversy, readers are referred to Biederman et al.[16]

1.2 Comorbidity

Researchers have attempted to distinguish between ADHD, bipolar disorder and combinations of the two. Some studies have reported comorbidity rates of ADHD ranging from 69 to 98% in children and adolescents with bipolar disorder.[19,25] Conversely, rates of bipolar disorder in children with ADHD are lower. Biederman at al.[15] reported that of 140 children (aged 6 to 17 years) diagnosed with ADHD by structured interviews, 11% had bipolar disorder at baseline and an additional 12% developed mania in the ensuing 4 years.

The high comorbidity rate may be related to overlapping symptoms. Biederman et al.[15] used proportional methods to control for 3 principal overlapping symptoms (distractibility, talkativeness and motoric overactivity), but no adjustment was made for other symptoms such as impulsivity, and the chronicity criteria of symptoms was not applied.

Kovacs and Pollock[26] reported a 69% lifetime comorbidity rate of conduct disorder in youths with bipolar disorder in a longitudinal study of psychiatrically referred patients. In the majority of these patients, conduct disorder with or without ADHD predated the affective episodes. This highlights the possibility of overlooking the onset of a bipolar disorder in chronically disruptive children.

In an epidemiological study, Carlson and Kashani[27] stated that 13% of adolescents from the general population who endorsed manic symptoms on diagnostic interviews were also found to have symptoms in virtually every other domain of psychopathology, including conduct disorder, behaviour disorder, anxiety disorder, depression and psychosis.

Epidemiological comorbidity studies of adults which include older adolescents indicate that substance use disorders may be more common in patients with bipolar disorder than in any other diagnostic group except conduct/antisocial personality disorders.[28,29] Less is known about the specificity of such an association in younger adolescents or children, although epidemiological studies find very high rates of mood and conduct comorbidity in substance-using adolescents.[30-32]

1.3 Differential Diagnosis

Many authors who have reported childhood mania have noted that the quality of affective symptoms does not always follow the typical pattern of that in adults.[10,33] Irritability, affective storminess and prolonged or extreme aggressive behaviours are perhaps as commonly described in children as euphoria, grandiosity or elated mood. In a group of children and adolescents with early-onset bipolar disorder and high rates of hyperactivity and mixed features, Geller et al.[34] reported very high rates of rapid-cycling features, where manic episodes may be of less than a week in duration but occur frequently. The presence of such a mixed picture may create difficulty distinguishing disruptive behaviour disorders, in which symptoms are typically chronic, from true mania. A careful longitudinal history is imperative to disentangle these issues.

Medical disorders such as encephalitis, syphilis, acquired immune deficiency states and hyperthyroidism must be ruled out. Neurological conditions such as trauma and seizure, and, less commonly (in this age group), multiple sclerosis, cerebritis in autoimmune disorders, right-sided cerebrovascular accidents and brain tumours may produce symptoms of mania. Administration of corticosteroids may also produce manic symptoms and there are some reported cases of antidepressants triggering mania (see section 3.3.3).

Alternative psychiatric disorders need be considered in the differential diagnosis of bipolar disorder. These include ADHD, conduct disorder, substance abuse and dependence, schizophrenia, schizoaffective disorder, agitated depression and post-traumatic stress disorder.

There are a number of approaches that help differentiate these conditions, including age of onset and course of illness. Symptoms of ADHD begin at an early age. In contrast, bipolar disorder most frequently occurs in mid-adolescence. Symptoms of ADHD are usually chronic and do not show improvement without treatment. In children with mania, the presenting symptoms are a distinct change from their usual behaviour. When examined systematically, classical manic symptoms (including elevated mood, increased sexual interest, pressured speech, grandiosity and racing thoughts) distinguish bipolar disorder from ADHD, while activity level and irritability do not.[35] Children with mania may have psychotic symptoms which are not a usual part of the ADHD constellation. Similarly, while patients often manifest serious misconduct during manic episodes, conduct disorder as an entity does not include symptoms of psychosis, delusional grandiosity, pressured speech or flight of ideas.

Bipolar disorder, especially in its early onset form, is often misdiagnosed as schizophrenia. Werry et al.,[36] in a systematic follow-up of 59 patients who presented with psychosis from ages 7 to 17 years, found that 23 met full criteria for bipolar disorder, although over half of these patients had initially been misdiagnosed as having schizophrenia. There may be different premorbid presentations that can be helpful in distinguishing patients with these two conditions. Patients with schizophrenia may have socially isolative traits with bizarre behaviour whereas patients with bipolar disorder may present with symptoms more suggestive of disruptive behaviour disorders with mood symptoms. Illness onset tends to be acute in children with mania as compared with a more insidious course in schizophrenia. Family history may also identify certain risk factors for either disorder.

Clinicians treating depressed children should be alert to the possibility that what presents initially as a unipolar illness may later switch to bipolarity. Geller et al.,[37] following 79 children initially diagnosed with major depression between the ages of 6 and 12 years, found that 32% developed manic (n = 10) or hypomanic (n = 15) episodes within 2 to 5 years. The only significant predictors of bipolar-I disorder were having 3 or more first- or second-degree relatives with major affective disorders and the early presence of bullying or fighting.

2. Epidemiology and Aetiology

In retrospective studies of adults with bipolar disorder, approximately 0.3 to 0.5% reported onset of symptoms before age 10 years of age,[2] in congruence with Kraepelin's[2] original description.

In an epidemiological study, Lewinsohn et al.[38] described a sample of 1709 adolescent patients and reported a lifetime prevalence of 1% (n = 18) for bipolar disorder. Carlson and Kashani,[27] in another epidemiological study of 14- to 16-year-old patients, reported the lifetime prevalence of mania to be less than 1%, which is congruent with epidemiological studies of adults worldwide.[39] No epidemiological studies have been conducted specifically to study the prevalence rates of prepubertal mania. Recent systematic population-based studies of childhood disorders have not found mania in pre-adolescents,[16] which lends support to the view that it is very rare.

Although the aetiology of bipolar disorder is unknown, the evidence from twin[40] and adoptive parent[41] studies suggest that there is a substantial genetic contribution.

3. Treatment

This section focuses on psychopharmacological interventions and the medical literature which supports their use. However, it should be kept in mind that pharmacotherapy is only one component of treatment. Optimal treatment consists of individualised planning for each patient. This includes incorporating psychosocial treatments, such as interpersonal therapy,[42] cognitive behavioural therapy[43] and even day treatment programmes that integrate a number of different modalities into the treatment plan.[44]

Clinicians should be alert to comorbid psychiatric conditions. The management of comorbid disorders should be geared at treating both disorders with a single effective agent, whenever possible. Attention needs to be focused on serious risk-taking behaviours such as suicide[45] that may occur in over 20% of adolescents with bipolar disorder, as well as substance abuse and risky sexual behaviour.[7] Family issues, including parents who may have undiagnosed bipolar disorder,[7] require attention and treatment. Finally, intervention of contributing or underlying medical illness is warranted.

Given that this discussion of the pharmacological management of mania and depression in children and adolescents is a brief overview, readers are referred to other sources for a more detailed discussion of specific clinic management issues.[46,47]

3.1 General Considerations

Despite years of clinic work in childhood bipolar disorder, there is a relative dearth of controlled studies on the efficacy of psychopharmacological interventions. There are child studies that report on the use of antimanic agents that are effective in adult forms of bipolar disorder, but in children their use has focused primarily on other disorders. Studies that have been published can be divided into three areas: (i) case reports;[48-53] (ii) open label studies;[54-56] and (iii) double-blind trials.[22,57-60] The adult literature on the other hand does demonstrate the efficacy of antimanic drugs, and consists of (uncontrolled) data on the potential efficacy of other medication groups as well.

It is useful to consider the treatment of bipolar disorder as consisting of two distinct phases: (i) acute management of mania or psychotic symptoms, usually requiring inpatient care; and (ii) the outpatient maintenance management between manic episodes.

Acute mania is best managed with antimanic agents as described in section 3.2, with adjunctive short term use of tranquillising medications (e.g. antipsychotics or benzo-diazepines) if agitation and insomnia are severe. Because children vary greatly in size and their ability to metabolise medications, the dosage guidelines outlined in sections 3.2 and 3.3 may need to be adjusted for smaller and younger children. It is wise to start low and titrate up to an ideal dosage as tolerated to minimise adverse effects and maximise compliance.

Once mania has remitted, the goal should be treatment with as few agents as possible to prevent relapse. Antidepressant medications may be necessary when depressive episodes occur.

3.2 Antimanic Agents

3.2.1 Lithium

Efficacy

Although lithium has been extensively studied in adults with bipolar disorder and in controlled trials for aggressive behaviour in children,[23] the majority of reports of its use in children and adolescents with bipolar disorder have been case presentations[7,51] and un-controlled open label trials.[54]

There has been only one double-blind trial of lithium in adolescents with bipolar disorder.[57] This was a placebo-controlled study of 25 adolescents who were diagnosed with a substance abuse disorder comorbid with a variety of mood disorders, either bipolar I, bipolar II or major depression with 'predictors' of bipolar disorder (bipolar disorder in a first degree relative, marked psychomotor retardation and/or switching to bipolar disorder during tricyclic anti-depressant treatment). Lithium resulted in a significant improvement in Clinical Global Assessment Scale scores and 6 of 13 patients (46%) were considered responders to lithium as compared with 1 of 12 patients who were considered responders to placebo.

In general, open label trials show response rates of around 65% with lithium. Despite evidence of short term efficacy, maintenance treatment with lithium has been reported to result in relapse in 37.5% of adolescents.[61] Lithium resistance has been seen in certain subgroups. These include those having an Axis I diagnosis before the age of 12 years,[62] comorbidity with a personality disorder,[63] and mixed or rapid cycling states.[64] This suggests that early onset or severe forms of bipolar disorder may be more difficult to treat.

Dosage

Lithium has a shorter half-life in children compared with adults.[65] Starting dosages can be effectively predicted based on bodyweight, approximately 30 mg/kg/day. This translates into starting dosages of 600 mg/day for children less than 25kg, and 900 mg/day for larger children. Using bodyweight to calculate initial dosages was found to be equivalent to more complicated repeated measurements in kinetics studies.[66] It should be kept in mind that lithium citrate may result in higher blood concentrations than carbonate preparations.[49]

Adverse Effects

Common adverse effects to lithium in children are similar to those experienced by adults and include bodyweight gain, tiredness, tremor, ataxia, dystonia, diplopia, polyuria, poly-dypsia, nausea and vomiting.[67] Adverse effects seem to be dose-related, but can occur at optimal as well as suboptimal therapeutic doses.

Acne is a possible adverse effect[68] which adolescents find distressing. Similarly, children and adolescents may be very embarrassed in school and community settings by tremor and bodyweight gain and may refuse to continue medication when they occur.

Thyroid enlargement[69] and elevated levels of thyroid stimulating hormone[70] have been reported in children, but were not accompanied by clinical hypothyroidism, as is occasionally reported in adults.[71] The issue of effects on thyroid function is complicated by reports indicating high rates of thyroid abnormalities in patients with mood disorders prior to medication exposure.[72]

The literature is mixed as to whether lithium impairs cognitive functioning in children.[60] Although the literature on adult patients treated with lithium discusses the possibility of renal impairment with long term use, this has not been reported in adolescents or children.[73] Another controversy in the adult literature is the risk of fetal malformations, with the consensus being that the use of lithium during pregnancy is association with some risk.[74]

Monitoring

Assessment of serum lithium concentrations should be performed on a regular basis; weekly for the first month, then monthly for 3 months, then as clinically indicated. Since controlled studies on therapeutic concentrations for children are lacking, practitioners should proceed with the assumption that blood concentrations need to be in the same range as those for adults, usually 0.8 to 1.2 mmol/L. Although the assessment of lithium concentrations using saliva has been investigated,[75] its clinical use is not recommended.

In addition, complete blood count (CBC), blood chemistries and thyroid function tests should be done at baseline, 1 month after starting medication and at least every 12 months thereafter. More stringent monitoring is needed in hot climates, and during fevers, excess sweating and exercise. Adequate fluid intake should be strongly encouraged.

Special Considerations

Lithium should be considered the first-line drug for childhood bipolar disorder, since it has been the most rigorously studied agent. An early onset of a psychiatric disorder may be associated with increased severity of illness. Since some children may have less than optimum responses to lithium, the need for alternative medications or combinations of medications must be made on an individual basis. The possibility of hypothyroidism and changes in renal function should be kept in mind. Laboratory testing for pregnancy should also be considered before starting and during treatment.

3.2.2 Valproic Acid (Sodium Valproate)

Efficacy

No controlled studies have been conducted using valproic acid (sodium valproate) in psychiatrically disordered youths, although the drug appears to be comparable in efficacy with lithium in adults with bipolar disorder.[76] Open studies support the use of the drug in children with disruptive behaviour[55] and bipolar disorder.[54,77] No information is available on its efficacy relative to lithium in this age group.

Dosage

As with adults, it is expected that an appropriate dosage of valproic acid in children is one that results in blood concentrations in the range of 50 to 100 mg/L. In practice, the starting dosage should be 250mg twice daily, with a suggested range between 1000 and 3000 mg/day.

Adverse Effects

Adverse effects associated with valproic acid include bodyweight gain, nausea and sedation. The adverse effects of the drug may be fewer and easier to tolerate for adolescents than those caused by lithium, resulting in better compliance.[78]

However, younger children are at risk for fatal hepatotoxicity. This risk is highest for children under the age of 2 years, and diminishes to close to zero after age 10 years.[79] Children receiving concomitant agents, especially other anticonvulsants, may also be at increased risk for liver damage. Concomitant use of lithium may increase bodyweight and cause gastro-intestinal complaints.

Of special concern in a study of 238 women receiving valproic acid for epilepsy, 89% of the adolescents in the study were reported to develop polycystic ovary disease, as opposed to 27% of adolescents receiving other medications.[80] Whether polycystic ovary disease is associated specifically with valproic acid for all patients or represents an effect specific to those with epilepsy is unclear.[81]

Monitoring

Certain adverse effects of valproic acid may be dose related. Consequently, blood concentrations should be assessed on a regular basis. For safety reasons, the range should be between 0.5 to 1.0 mg/L. Because of the risk of hepatotoxicity, baseline blood work should be done and followed by assessments at 1-month intervals for the first 6 months, and every 6 months thereafter. Monitoring should include CBC with differential, routine blood chemistries and liver function tests.

Special Considerations

Valproic acid may be better tolerated by children than lithium. However, the combination of less systematic attention to this compound in children and the risk of hepatotoxicity suggest that valproic acid should be considered a second-line agent in childhood bipolar disorder.

3.2.3 Carbamazepine

Efficacy

Carbamazepine may be helpful in children and adolescents with bipolar disorder but little systematic research has been devoted to this compound. It has been used primarily as adjunctive treatment in children with lithium-resistant disorder.[82] As with lithium and valproic acid, carbamazepine has been used in children with a variety of other disorders, including aggression associated with conduct disorder, and with mixed results.[56,58]

Dosage

The starting dosage should be 100 to 200mg per day, with increasing increments of 50mg every 2 to 3 days if possible. Maintenance dosages may range from 400 to 600 mg/day, as long as blood concentrations remain below 12 mg/L.

Adverse Effects

Common adverse effects associated with carbamazepine include dizziness, nausea, vomiting and sedation. In particular, the drug is known to cause behavioural toxicity,[56] so that a child's behaviour can actually worsen rather than improve while they are receiving this medication. There is also a risk of aplastic anaemia or agranulocytosis, liver toxicity and rashes.

Monitoring

Therapeutic carbamazepine concentrations for seizure disorders are usually reported to be in the range of 4 to 12 mg/L. Weekly CBC with differential and platelets should be performed during the first month, then monthly for 3 months, and then as clinically indicated. Blood chemistries and liver function tests should be assessed at baseline, repeated at 1 and 3 months, and then at least every 12 months.

Special Considerations

It is unclear how efficacious carbamazepine is as monotherapy in patients with bipolar disorder; therefore, it should be considered a second-line agent. Serious adverse effects have been related to carbamazepine use and it produces 'auto-induction' of hepatic enzymes, which can be expected to peak at 4 to 6 weeks, requiring dosage adjustment over that period.[83]

3.2.4 Antipsychotics

Efficacy

A modestly sized study suggested that lithium alone can effectively treat psychotic symptoms as well as manic symptoms in children.[84] However, a study currently under way has reported that adolescents with psychotic bipolar disorder may require the addition of an antipsychotic to lithium to control psychotic symptoms.[85]

Haloperidol has been used in various disruptive disorders, in particular in aggression associated with conduct disorder;[22] however, adverse effects occur which may contribute to compliance difficulties.[22]

Studies in adults are beginning to produce evidence that low doses of the novel antipsychotic agents, risperidone and olanzapine, are effective at controlling bipolar symptoms.[86,87] Case reports support the use of low-dose risperidone in adolescents with bipolar disorder.[50] Clozapine was reported to be effective in one adolescent with bipolar disorder,[88] but because of the risk of agranulocytosis, which can occur at any time during the course of treatment, it should not be considered a first-line agent.

Dosage

It appears that dosages (2 mg/day risperidone and 5 mg/day olanzapine) approximately half those employed to treat psychotic symptoms are being used to treat the symptoms of bipolar disorder in adults. Case studies of adolescents and children suggest using lower dosages (0.25mg risperidone twice daily). Our clinical experience with olanzapine in pre-adolescents with bipolar disorder is that 5mg or more per day is prohibitively sedating. Clozapine dosages above 300 mg/day are also likely to result in significant adverse effects.

Adverse Effects

Traditional antipsychotics have significant adverse effects that may interfere with compliance. These include bodyweight gain, sedation, extrapyramidal symptoms (EPS) and movement disorders, including tardive dyskinesia. EPS tend to occur less frequently with risperidone and olanzapine than with the typical antipsychotics, although sedation and bodyweight gain continue to be significant problems with these newer agents. The atypical agents are suggested to be less likely to cause tardive dyskinesia. Sedation is a particular problem in that it interferes with academic functioning.

Neuroleptic malignant syndrome, although rare, is a potentially fatal adverse effect.[89] All antipsychotics can cause hyperprolactinaemia, galactorrhoea and interruption of normal menses, although it is believed that atypicals are less likely to cause these effects than typical agents.

Monitoring

Blood concentrations do not appear to provide useful clinical information for either typical or atypical agents. Laboratory work ups (CBC and blood chemistries) and electrocardiograms should be obtained at baseline and at 12-month intervals in patients receiving typical or atypical antipsychotics. Dispensing of clozapine requires (in the US) white blood cell counts (WBC) every 2 weeks for the whole of the treatment period. If baseline WBC is less than 3500 WBC/mm^2, clozapine should not be initiated. During treatment, levels of 3000 to 3500 WBC/mm^2 require twice weekly WBC counts, and below 3000 WBC/mm^2 clozapine should be discontinued.

Special Considerations

Antipsychotic-induced abnormal movements are always a potential risk and formal assessments performed every 3 months are clinically indicated.[90] The occurrence of adverse effects with antipsychotics should be monitored for, as they frequently contribute to compliance problems.

3.3 Other Medications and Somatic Treatments

3.3.1 Other Anticonvulsants

Gabapentin[91] and lamotrigine[92] are beginning to be investigated in the treatment of bipolar disorder in adults. However, no studies of the use of these agents in this indication in children have been performed. Furthermore, the risk of life-threatening rashes, including Stevens-Johnson Syndrome, can occur in adolescents and children exposed to lamotrigine. In the US, lamotrigine is not approved for use in children under the age of 16 years. Gabapentin has been reported to worsen aggressive behaviour in some children being treated for seizures.[93]

3.3.2 Stimulants

Because of the overlap between ADHD and bipolar symptoms in children (see sections 1.1.1 and 1.2), stimulants have often been prescribed prior to the diagnosis of bipolar disorder. One case report has suggested that methylphenidate may worsen symptoms of bipolar disorder.[94] Conversely, an adolescent with brain injury who met the criteria for bipolar disorder reportedly responded only to dexamphetamine (dextroamphetamine).[95]

A placebo-controlled study of methylphenidate plus lithium[96] examined the effect of these medications on ADHD symptoms in 7 children with ADHD comorbid with various other disorders, including mania. Little clinical benefit was seen from either medication alone or the combination, although the small sample size limits the generalisability of this study.

3.3.3 Antidepressants

Although antidepressants have been in common usage clinically in child psychiatry for many years, controlled studies of these agents for the treatment of major depression in children and adolescents have generally failed to demonstrate superiority over placebo until recently. A large systematic study of fluoxetine in children and adolescents[97] and a recently completed multicentre trial of paroxetine in adolescents (R. Klein, personal communication) have shown that these selective serotonin (5-hydroxytryptamine; 5-HT) reuptake inhibitors (SSRIs) are more effective than placebo in the treatment of depression in this population. Although these studies excluded patients with known bipolar illness, it is presumed that, as in adults, treatments efficacious for unipolar depression should also be effective in bipolar depression.

However, clinicians should be aware of the potential risk of triggering a manic episode. While there are many case reports of the onset of mania while children or adolescents were receiving antidepressant medication,[98,99] the issue of whether antidepressants cause mania in youths has received inadequate systematic study. SSRIs[100] and tricyclic antidepressants[98,99] have been associated with such a conversion, but statistically controlled analysis of systematic follow-up has not demonstrated that exposure to antidepressants increases the rate of onset of mania in children to a greater extent than placebo treatment.[37,101] Nonetheless, clinical wisdom warrants using mood-stabilisers in conjunction with antidepressants in patients who have had previous manic episodes.

3.3.4 Electroconvulsive Therapy
Electroconvulsive therapy (ECT) has been described as effective in 2 children with refractory bipolar disorder.[102] However, this treatment should be considered only in those severe cases where all other interventions have failed.

3.3.5 Multiple Medications
Clinicians are frequently faced with patients whose symptoms have responded poorly to monotherapy. In these instances, combinations of medications may need consideration. In particular, adding an anticonvulsant to lithium may increase the response rate. Two reports support the combination of lithium plus valproic acid in children with refractory bipolar disorder.[54,103]

High potency benzodiazepines are frequently used adjunctively to manage severe agitation and insomnia during the acute treatment of mania, although there are no controlled studies in children supporting the safety or efficacy of this approach. Because of the potential for abuse and dependence, as well as the disinhibiting effect in children, these drugs should be used only cautiously and briefly.

Individual patients have been reported to respond to the addition of other medications to the standard regimen. Thyroxine (levothyroxine) at a dosage of 125 μg/day was used effectively as an adjunct to valproic acid in a 13-year-old male who had normal thyroid functions and treatment-resistant, rapid-cycling bipolar disorder.[48] The rationale for such an approach is based upon high rates of thyroid-axis abnormalities, in the absence of clinical thyroid disorders, found in adults and adolescents with affective disorders.[72]

Although there have been mixed reports of the antimanic effects of verapamil in adults,[104] one adolescent with mental retardation and a complicated behavioural picture responded to a combination of valproic acid and verapamil.[52] Melatonin plus alprazolam was reportedly effective in another case.[105]

Any decision to combine agents should take into account drug interactions, including metabolism involving the cytochrome P450 system, and the impact on plasma protein binding affinity, which can drastically affect blood drug concentrations.

4. Conclusion
Bipolar disorder is an uncommon disorder in childhood. The diagnostic criteria applied should be similar to those used in adults, incorporating developmental differences where appropriate. There is little systematic research on the treatment of this disorder in childhood and further empirical investigation is warranted. However, lithium seems to be the first-line treatment for this disorder. It should be kept in mind that psychopharmacological intervention is only one facet of the treatment for this disorder.

References

1. Esquirol E. Mental maladies. A treatise of insanity. Philadelphia (PA): Lea and Blanchard Philadelphia, 1845
2. Goodwin F, Jamison K. Manic depressive illness. New York (NY): Oxford University Press, 1990
3. Berrios GE. Depressive and manic states during the nineteenth century. In: Georgotas A, Cancro R, editors. Depression and mania. New York (NY): Elsevier Science Publishing Co., 1988: 13-25
4. Biederman J, Wozniak J, Kiely K, et al. CBCL clinical scales discriminate prepubertal children with structured interview-derived diagnosis of mania from those with ADHD. J Am Acad Child Adolesc Psychiatry 1995; 34: 464-71
5. Wozniak J, Biederman J, Mundy E, et al. A pilot family study of childhood-onset mania. J Am Acad Child Adolesc Psychiatry 1995; 34: 1577-83
6. Birmaher B, Ryan ND, Williamson D, et al. Child and adolescent depression: a review of the past 10 years. Part I. J Am Acad Child Adolesc Psychiatry 1997; 35: 1427-39
7. Geller B, Luby J. Child and adolescent bipolar disorder: a review of the past 10 years. J Am Acad Child Adolesc Psychiatry 1997; 36: 1168-76
8. Hechtman L, Greenfield B. Juvenile onset bipolar disorder. Curr Opin Paediatr 1997; 9: 346-53
9. McClellan J, Werry J. Practice parameters for the assessment and treatment of children and adolescents with bipolar disorder. J Am Acad Child Adolesc Psychiatry 1997; 36: 157S-176S
10. Weller EB, Weller RA, Fristad MA. Bipolar disorder in children: misdiagnosis, underdiagnosis, and future directions. J Am Acad Child Adolesc Psychiatry 1995; 34: 709-14
11. American Psychiatric Association. Diagnostic and statistical manual of mental disorders. 4th ed. Washington, DC: American Psychiatric Association, 1994
12. McElroy SL, Strakowski SM, West SA, et al. Phenomenology of adolescent and adult mania in hospitalised patients with bipolar disorder. Am J Psychiatry 1997; 154: 44-9
13. Keck PE, McElroy SL, Strakowski SM, et al. 12-month outcome of patients with bipolar disorder following hospitalisation for a manic or mixed episode. Am J Psychiatry 1998; 155; 646-52
14. Akiskal HS. Developmental pathways to bipolarity: are juvenile-onset depressions pre-bipolar?. J Am Acad Child Adolesc Psychiatry 1995; 34 (6): 754-63
15. Biederman J, Faraone S, Mick E, et al. Attention-deficit hyperactivity disorder and juvenile mania: an overlooked comorbidity? J Am Acad Child Adolesc Psychiatry 1996; 35 (8): 997-1008
16. Biederman J, Klein R, Pine DS, et al. Resolved: mania is mistaken for ADHD in prepubertal children. J Am Acad Child Adolesc Psychiatry 1998; 37: 1091-9
17. Faraone SV, Biederman J, Mennin D, et al. Attention-deficit hyperactivity disorder with bipolar disorder: a familial subtype? J Am Acad Child Adolesc Psychiatry 1997; 36: 1378-90
18. West SA, McElroy SL, Strakowski SM, et al. Attention deficit hyperactivity disorder in adolescent mania. Am J Psychiatry 1995; 152: 271-3
19. Wozniak J, Biederman J, Kiely K, et al. Mania-like symptoms suggestive of childhood-onset bipolar disorder in clinically referred children. J Am Acad Child Adolesc Psychiatry 1995; 34: 867-76
20. Winokur G, Coryell W, Endicott J, et al. Further distinctions between manic-depressive illness (bipolar disorder) and primary depressive disorder (unipolar depression). Am J Psychiatry 1993; 150: 1176-81
21. Campbell M, Fish B, Korien J, et al. Lithium and chlorpromazine: a controlled crossover study of hyperactive severely disturbed young children. J Autism Child Schizophr 1972; 2: 234-63
22. Campbell M, Small AM, Green WH, et al. Behavioural efficacy of haloperidol and lithium carbonate. Arch Gen Psychiatry 1984; 41: 650-6
23. Campbell M, Kafantaris V, Cueva JE. An update on the use of lithium carbonate in aggressive children and adolescents with conduct disorder. Psychopharmacol Bull 1995; 31 (1): 93-102
24. Bradley C. The behaviour of children receiving benzedrine. Am J Psychiatry 1937; 94: 577-85
25. West SA, Strakowski SM, Sax KW, et al. The comorbidity of attention-deficit hyperactivity disorder in adolescent mania: potential diagnostic and treatment implications. Psychopharmacol Bull 1995; 31: 347-51
26. Kovacs M, Pollock M. Bipolar disorder and comorbid conduct disorder in childhood and adolescence. J Am Acad Child Adolesc Psychiatry 1995; 34 (6): 715-23
27. Carlson GA, Kashani JH. Manic symptoms in a non-referred adolescent population. J Affect Disord 1988; 15: 219-26
28. Kessler RC, Nelson CB, McGonagle KA, et al. The epidemiology of co-occurring addictive and mental disorders: implications for prevention and service utilisation. Am J Orthopsychiatry 1996; 66: 17-31
29. Regier DA, Farmer ME, Rae DS, et al. Comorbidity of mental disorders with alcohol and other drug abuse. Results from the Epidemiologic Catchment Area (ECA) Study. JAMA 1990; 264 (19): 2511-8
30. Boyle MH, Offord DR. Psychiatric disorder and substance use in adolescence. Can J Psychiatry 1991; 36: 699-705
31. Fergusson DM, Horwood LJ, Lynsky MT. Prevalence and comorbidity of DSM-III-R diagnoses in a birth cohort of 15 year olds. J Am Acad Child Adolesc Psychiatry 1993; 32: 28-33
32. Kandel DB, Johnson JG, Birdh, et al. Psychiatric disorders associated with substance use among children and adolescents: findings from the Methods for the Epidemiology of Child and Adolescent Mental Disorders (MECA) Study. J Abnorm Child Psychol 1997; 25 (2): 121-32
33. Carlson GA. Identifying prepubertal mania. J Am Acad Child Adolesc Psychiatry 1995; 34: 750-3
34. Geller B, Sun K, Zimerman B, et al. Complex and rapid-cycling in bipolar children and adolescents: a preliminary study. J Affect Disord 1995; 34 (4): 259-68
35. Fristad MA, Weller EB, Weller RA. The Mania Rating Scale: can it be used in children? A preliminary report. J Am Acad Child Adolesc Psychiatry 1992; 31 (2): 252-7

36. Werry JS, McClellan JM, Chard L. Childhood adolescent schizophrenic, bipolar, and schizoaffective disorders: a clinical and outcome study. J Am Acad Child Adolesc Psychiatry 1991; 30 (3): 457-65
37. Geller B, Fox LW, Clark KA. Rate and predictors of prepubertal bipolarity during follow-up of 6- to 12-year-old depressed children. J Am Acad Child Adolesc Psychiatry 1994; 33 (4): 461-8
38. Lewinsohn PM, Klein DN, Seeley JR. Bipolar disorders in a community sample of older adolescents: prevalence, phenomenology, comorbidity, and course. J Am Acad Child Adolesc Psychiatry 1995; 34: 454-63
39. Weissman MM, Bland RC, Canino GJ, et al. Cross-national epidemiology of major depression and bipolar disorder. JAMA 1996; 276 (4): 293-9
40. Nurnberger JI, Gershon E. Genetics. In: Paykel ES, editor. Handbook of affective disorders. 1st ed. New York (NY): Churchill-Livingstone, 1982
41. Mendlewicz J, Rainer JD. Adoption study supporting genetic transmission in manic depressive illness. Nature 1977; 265: 327-9
42. Mufson L, Fairbanks J. Interpersonal psychotherapy for depressed adolescents: a one year follow-up study. J Am Acad Child Adolesc Psychiatry 1996; 35: 1145-55
43. Goldman EL. CBT: a healing odyssey for bipolar patients. Clinical Psychiatry News 1998 Sep: 27
44. Matzner FJ, Silvan M, Silva RR, et al. Intensive day program for disturbed truant adolescents. Am J Orthopsychiatry 1998; 68: 135-41
45. Strober M, Schmidt-Lackner S, Freeman R, et al. Recovery and relapse in adolescents with bipolar affective illness: a five-year naturalistic, prospective follow-up. J Am Acad Child Adolesc Psychiatry 1995; 34: 724-31
46. Kutcher S. Child and adolescent psychopharmacology. Philadelphia (PA): W.B. Saunders Co., 1997
47. Walsh BT, editor. Child psychopharmacology. Washington, DC: American Psychiatric Press, Inc., 1998
48. Weeston TF, Constantino J. High-dose T4 for rapid-cycling bipolar disorder [letter]. J Am Acad Child Adolesc Psychiatry 1996; 35: 131-2
49. Reisher H, Pfeffer C. Lithium pharmacokinetics. J Am Acad Child Adolesc Psychiatry 1996; 35: 130-1
50. Fras I, Major LF. Clinical experience with risperidone [letter]. J Am Acad Child Adolesc Psychiatry 1995; 34: 833
51. Samuel RZ. EPS with lithium [letter]. J Am Acad Child Adolesc Psychiatry 1993; 32: 1078
52. Kastner T, Friedman DL. Verapamil and valproic acid treatment of prolonged mania. J Am Acad Child Adolesc Psychiatry 1992; 31: 271-5
53. Shliselberg N, Bosch JR, Herrera J. Valproic acid in the treatment of refractory bipolar disorder [letter]. J Clin Psychopharmacol 1990; 10: 151-2
54. Kafantaris V, Dicker R, Coletti DJ, et al. Combined lithium and divalproex treatment of bipolar adolescents: an open pilot study. Poster presentation, New Clinical Drug Evaluation Unit 38th Annual Meeting: 1998 Jun 9-12; Boca Raton, Florida
55. Donovan S, Susser ES, Nunes EV, et al. Divalproex treatment of disruptive adolescents: a report of 10 cases. J Clin Psychiatry 1997; 58: 12-5
56. Kafantaris V, Campbell M, Padron-Gayol MV, et al. Carbamazepine in hospitalised aggressive conduct disorder children: an open pilot study. Psychopharmacol Bull 1992; 28: 193-9
57. Geller B, Cooper TB, Sun K, et al. Double-blind and placebo-controlled study of lithium for adolescent bipolar disorders with secondary substance dependency. J Am Acad Child Adolesc Psychiatry 1998; 37: 171-8
58. Cueva JE, Overall JE, Small AM, et al. Carbamazepine in aggressive children with conduct disorder: a double-blind placebo-controlled study. J Am Acad Child Psychiatry 1996; 35 (4): 480-90
59. Campbell M, Adams PB, Small AM, et al. Lithium in hospitalised aggressive children with conduct disorder: a double-blind and placebo controlled study. J Acad Child Adolesc Psychiatry 1995; 34: 445-53
60. Silva RR, Campbell M, Golden RR, et al. Side effects associated with lithium and placebo administration in aggressive children. Psychopharmacol Bull 1992; 28: 319-26
61. Strober M, Morrell W, Lampert C, et al. Relapse following discontinuation of lithium maintenance therapy in adolescents with bipolar I illness: a naturalistic study. Am J Psychiatry 1990; 147: 457-61
62. Strober M, Lampert C, Schmidt S, et al. The course of major depressive disorder in adolescents: I. Recovery and risk of manic switching in a follow-up of psychotic and nonpsychotic subtypes. J Am Acad Child Adolesc Psychiatry 1993; 32: 34-42
63. Kutcher SP, Marton P, Korenblum M. Adolescent bipolar illness and personality disorder. J Am Acad Child Adolesc Psychiatry 1990; 29: 355-8
64. Prien RF, Potter WZ. NIMH workshop report on treatment of bipolar disorder. Psychopharmacol Bull 1990; 26: 409-27
65. Vitiello B, Behar D, Malone R, et al. Pharmacokinetics of lithium carbonate in children. J Clin Psychopharmacol 1988; 8: 355-9
66. Hagino OR, Weller EB, Weller RA, et al. Comparison of lithium dosage methods for preschool- and early school-age children. J Am Acad Child Adolesc Psychiatry 1998; 37: 60-5
67. Campbell M, Silva RR, Kafantaris V, et al. Predictors of side effects associated with lithium administration in children. Psychopharmacol Bull 1991; 27: 373-80
68. Lapierre YD, Raval KJ. Pharmacotherapy of affective disorders in children and adolescents. Psychiatr Clin North Am 1989; 12: 951-61
69. DeLong GR, Aldershof AL. Long-term experience with lithium treatment in childhood: correlation with clinical diagnosis. J Am Acad Child Adolesc Psychiatry 1987; 26: 389-94
70. Picker W, Solomon G, Gertner JM. Lithium side effect [letter]. J Am Acad Child Adolesc Psychiatry 1990; 29 (3): 489
71. Ortiz A, Dabbagh M, Gershon S. Lithium: clinical use, toxicology and mode of action. In: Bernstein JG, editor. Clinical psychopharmacology. 2nd ed. Littleton (MA): John Wright-PSG Inc., 1984

72. Sokolov ST, Kutcher SP, Joffe RT. Basal thyroid indices in adolescent depression and bipolar disorder. J Am Acad Child Adolesc Psychiatry 1994; 33 (4): 469-75
73. Kafantaris V. Treatment of bipolar disorder in children and adolescents. J Am Acad Child Adolesc Psychiatry 1995; 34: 732-41
74. Cohen LS, Friedman JM, Jefferson JW, et al. A reevaluation of risk of in utero exposure to lithium. JAMA 1994; 230: 1283-7
75. Weller EB, Weller RA, Fristad MA, et al. Saliva lithium monitoring in prepubertal children. J Am Acad Child Adolesc Psychiatry 1987; 26: 173-5
76. American Psychiatric Association. Practice guideline for the treatment of patients with bipolar disorder. Am J Psychiatry 1994; 151 (12 Suppl.): 1-36
77. Papatheodorou G, Kutcher SP, Katic M, et al. The efficacy and safety of divalproex sodium in the treatment of acute mania in adolescents and young adults: an open clinical trial. J Clin Psychopharmacol 1995; 15 (2): 110-6
78. McConville BJ, Sorter MT, Foster K, et al. Lithium versus valproate side effects in adolescents with bipolar disorder. Poster presentation New Clinical Drug Evaluation Unit 38th Annual Meeting: 1998 Jun 9-12; Boca Raton, Florida
79. Bryant III AE, Dreifuss FE. Valproic acid hepatic fatalities. Neurology 1996; 46: 465-9
80. Inojarvi JIT, Laatikainen TJ, Pakarinen AJ, et al. Polycystic ovaries and hyperandrogenism in women taking valproate for epilepsy. N Engl J Med 1993; 329: 1383-8
81. Irwin M, Masand P. Valproate and polycystic ovaries [letter]. J Am Acad Child Adolesc Psychiatry 1998; 37 (1): 9-10
82. Garfinkel M, Garfinkel L, Himmelhoch J, et al. Lithium carbonate and carbamazepine: an effective treatment for adolescent manic or mixed bipolar patients. Annual meeting of the American Academy of Child and Adolescent Psychiatry, 1985; 41-42
83. Silva RR, Munoz DM, Alpert M. Carbamazepine use in children and adolescents with features of attention deficit hyperactivity disorder. J Acad Child Adolesc Psychiatry 1996; 35: 352-8
84. Varanka TM, Weller RA, Weller EB, et al. Lithium treatment of manic episodes with psychotic features in prepubertal children. Am J Psychiatry 1988; 145: 1557-9
85. Kafantaris V, Coletti DJ, Dicker R, et al. Are childhood psychiatric histories of bipolar adolescents associated with family history, psychosis, and response to lithium treatment? J Affect Disord 1998; 51 (2): 153-64
86. Tohen M, Zarate CA. Antipsychotic agents and bipolar disorder. J Clin Psychiatry 1998; 59: 38-49
87. Sanger TM, Tohen M, Tollefson GD, et al. Olanzapine versus placebo in the treatment of acute mania [abstract]. Schizophrenia Res 1998; 29: 152
88. Fuchs DC. Clozapine treatment of bipolar disorder in a young adolescent. J Am Acad Child Adolesc Psychiatry 1994; 33: 1299-302
89. Silva RR, Alpert M, Munoz, DM, et al. Neuroleptic malignant syndrome in children and adolescents. J Am Acad Child Adolesc Psychiatry 1999; 38 (2): 187-94
90. Silva RR, Magee HJ, Friedhoff AJ. Persistent tardive dyskinesia and other neuroleptic related dyskinesias in tourette's disorder. J Child Adolesc Psychopharmacol 1993; 3: 137-44
91. McElroy SL, Soutullo CA, Keck PE, et al. A pilot trial of adjunctive gabapentin in treatment of bipolar disorder. Annals Clin Psychiatry 1997; 9: 99-103
92. Kusumakar V, Yatham L. Lamotrigine treatment of rapid cycling bipolar disorder [letter]. Am J Psychiatry 1997; 154: 1171-2
93. Lee DO, Steingard RJ, Cesena M, et al. Behavioural side effects of gabapentin in children. Epilepsia 1996; 37 (1): 87-90
94. Koehler-Troy C, Strober M, Malenbaum R. Methylphenidate-induced mania in a prepubertal child. J Clin Psychiatry 1986; 47: 566-7
95. Max JE, Richards L, Hamdan-Allen G. Case study: antimanic effectiveness of dextroamphetamine in a brain-injured adolescent. J Am Acad Child Adolesc Psychiatry 1995; 34 (4): 472-6
96. Carlson GA, Rapport MD, Kelly KL, et al. The effects of methylphenidate and lithium on attention and activity level. J Am Acad Child Adolesc Psychiatry 1992; 31: 262-70
97. Emslie GJ, Rush AJ, Weinberg WA, et al. A double-blind randomised, placebo-controlled trial of fluoxetine in children and adolescents with depression. Arch Gen Psychiatry 1997; 54 (11): 1031-7
98. Kashani JH, Hodges KK, Shekim WO. Hypomanic reaction to amityptyline in a depressed child. Psychosomatics 1980; 21 (10): 867, 872
99. Briscoe JJ, Harrington RC, Predergast M. Development of mania in close association with tricyclic antidepressant administration in children. A report of two cases. Eur Child Adolesc Psychiatry 1995; 4 (4): 280-3
100. Venkataraman S, Naylor MW, King CA. Mania associated with fluoxetine treatment in adolescents. J Am Acad Child Adolesc Psychiatry 1992; 31: 276-81
101. Geller B, Fox LW, Fletcher M. Effect of tricyclic antidepressants on switching to mania and on the onset of bipolarity in depressed 6 to 12 year olds. J Am Acad Child Adolesc Psychiatry 1993; 32: 43-50
102. Hill MA, Courvoisie H, Dawkins K, et al. ECT for the treatment of intractable mania in two prepubertal male children. Convuls Ther 1997; 13: 74-82
103. Hsu LK. Lithium-resistant adolescent mania. J Am Acad Child Psychiatry 1986; 25: 280-3
104. Barton B, Gitlin MJ. Verapamil in treatment-resistant mania: an open trial. J Clin Psychopharmacol 1987; 7: 101-3
105. Robertson JM, Tanguay PE. Case study: the use of melatonin in a boy with refractory bipolar disorder. J Am Acad Child Adolesc Psychiatry 1997; 36: 822-5

Correspondence: Dr *Raul R. Silva*, New York University School of Medicine, Division of Child and Adolescent Psychiatry, 550 First Avenue, Room NB2156, New York, NY 10019, USA.

Depression in Children and Adolescents

A Guide to Diagnosis and Treatment

Graham J. Emslie and *Taryn L. Mayes*

University of Texas Southwestern Medical Center at Dallas and Children's Medical Center of Dallas, Dallas, Texas, USA

Depressive disorders are leading causes of morbidity and mortality in the paediatric age group,[1-3] with a prevalence rate of up to 8.3%.[4] This prevalence is similar to that in adults,[5] and is greater in adolescents than children. Major depressive disorder (MDD) in children appears to occur at approximately the same rate in girls and boys, with the approximately 2 : 1 ratio becoming evident in adolescents.[6,7]

1. Diagnosis

1.1 Clinical Presentation

Children and adolescents do not generally refer themselves for treatment, and are brought for treatment because of problems that are not initially evident as depression. For example, depressed children will be referred because of nonspecific physical complaints (stomach aches, headaches, etc.) or because of negative irritable mood leading to oppositional behaviours and refusal to do school work or attend school. In adolescents, the presenting problem may be suicidal thoughts or behaviours or antisocial behaviour, including substance abuse. What makes the diagnostic process more challenging is the fact that when evaluated systematically, many children with depression meet criteria for other comorbid disorders, including anxiety disorders and disruptive disorders.[8] These comorbid conditions are not entirely a function of symptom overlap.

Important for the clinician to emphasise, however, is that depression is a diagnosable condition in this age group and does not have to be inferred from an array of behaviours. One of the major advances in clinical child psychiatry in the past 20 years is the recognition that internalising disorders (depression and anxiety) can be reliably diagnosed in this age group. The diagnostic criteria for depression are essentially the same for children, adolescents and adults,[9] except for the inclusion of irritable mood. The difference from adults is in the diagnostic process itself. Accurate diagnosis requires the use of multiple informants: child, parent, often school, and a clinician experienced in synthesising the information from multiple sources. An additional finding is that children are reliable reporters of some symptoms that are not well reported by parents, i.e. more internalising symptoms, including depressed mood, decreased interest and sleep, and appetite changes. This process of interviewing has been operationalised in research diagnostic interviews, such as the Kiddie Schedule for Affective Disorders and Schizophrenia – Present and Lifetime Version (K-SADS-PL),[10] which has been shown to have reliability and validity. While research diagnostic interviews are not used in clinical practice, some familiarity with them is helpful for clinicians wanting to improve their diagnostic acumen.

As assessment of depression in this age group requires information from multiple sources, self-report instruments have limited diagnostic utility, but can be a useful adjunct to assessment. Two self-report scales designed specifically for children are the Childhood Depression Inventory (CDI)[11] and the Weinberg Depression Scale for Children and Adolescents (WDSCA).[12]

1.2 Diagnostic Criteria

The three primary depressive disorders found in children and adolescents are MDD, dysthymic disorder and depressive disorder not otherwise specified (NOS).[9] MDD tends to be episodic, with either full or partial recovery between episodes. The episodes, which require at least 2 weeks of symptoms, cause significant impairment in the child's functioning, as evidenced by declined school performance, withdrawal and increased conflicts in relationships. Depressive disorder NOS (minor depression) is also episodic, but the number of symptoms, length of episode or impairment in functioning are not as severe as those in MDD.

Dysthymia is a chronic dysphoria that, although less intense than MDD, has no prolonged well states. Children may have good and bad days, but they do not have good weeks. Often these children have had symptoms since their preschool years. As they grow older, MDD often develops, which is called a 'double depression'. Studies by Kovacs et al.[13] in children and reports in adults[14] identify the long term disability evident in early onset dysthymic disorder. In the long term follow-up study by Kovacs et al.,[13] over 70% developed 'double depression' over the course of 5 years. Recent studies identify the increasing risk of suicide as children with chronic depression move into adolescence.[15,16]

1.3 Differential Diagnoses

As mentioned in section 1.1, the diagnosis of a mood disorder is often obscured by the presence of other comorbid psychiatric diagnoses. In fact, Puig-Antich et al.[17] suggest that "the search for 'pure' (i.e. non-comorbid) forms of very-early-onset affective illness may be a futile undertaking, as comorbidity may be an intrinsic characteristic of children with major affective illness and their families as well". Kovacs[15] has suggested that, compared with adults, children exhibit high rates of non-affective diagnoses, primarily anxiety disorders, behaviour disorder and substance abuse. In her sample of child/adolescent outpatients with MDD, 88% had concurrent non-affective diagnoses. Comorbidity of depression with general medical conditions is also frequent. Studies have identified high rates of psychiatric disorders in children and adolescents with various neurological conditions,[18,19] including brain injury,[20-22] epilepsy,[23-26] migraine[27] and learning disabilities.[28-32]

As differential diagnoses can at times be complex, a detailed family history can provide additional information, e.g. to aid in diagnosis and treatment decisions. The offspring of adults with affective illness show a high rate of depression and bipolar disorder.[14] Children with MDD have high familial aggregation of depression, alcoholism, anxiety and other psychiatric diagnoses in first- and second-degree relatives.[33,34] It has been noted that 50 to 80% of children and adolescents with MDD have a positive family history of mood disorders.

1.4 Clinical Course

MDD is an episodic disorder. Therefore, of interest is not only the overall outcome, but also the course of depressive symptoms during the intervening periods. Recovery from an index episode of major depression is remarkably consistent across samples, with over 90% of depressed child and adolescent outpatients,[13,35] child and adolescent inpatients[36,37] and nonreferred adolescents[38] having recovered from an episode of MDD within 1 to 2 years. In two of these samples,[13,39] recovery occurred with minimal treatment in the majority of patients. This is similar to findings in adults.[40,41]

Once recovered, depressed children and adolescents have a high rate of recurrence of their depression. When re-evaluated 6 to 7 years later, depression remained a problem in 40 to 50% of clinical patients[42-45] and in around 25% of nonreferred individuals identified by community sampling.[46,47] Recurrence (a new episode of depression) is reported in 54 to 72% of depressed children and adolescents followed for 3 to 8 years, with similar rates in inpatients[37,48] and outpatients.[8,16,35,49]

For some children and adolescents, depression continues into adult mood disorders. Harrington et al.,[50] in a retrospective follow-up study of 80 depressed and 80 nondepressed outpatient adolescents, showed that, as adults, depressive disorders were more common in the group who were depressed adolescents; however, they note that most adult depressions are not preceded by adolescent depression.

In summary, depression in children and adolescents is a diagnosable condition that still is frequently undetected. It is associated with increased family problems and school failure and, particularly in adolescents, suicide, substance abuse and truancy. Depression is often a chronic condition and needs to be identified early to maximise the potential for treatment. Overall, the phenomenology and biology (see Emslie et al.,[8] for review) of depression in children and adolescents are similar to those of adult depression. However, accurate diagnosis requires experience in the diagnostic assessment of children, given the difference in the diagnostic process.

2. Treatment

2.1 General Treatment Approach

Assessment of a child or adolescent with depression (or any psychiatric disorder) will include an assessment of psychosocial stressors, family functioning, school environment and an assessment of the individual's coping abilities. Frequently, it is difficult clinically to separate the factors that precipitate or maintain depressive symptoms from the consequences of the depression itself.

However, treatment will be focused towards both the precipitants and consequences of the depression and will be multimodal, including the child, parents and school. The primary aim of treatment is to shorten the episode of depression (remission), to prevent recurrence and to decrease the negative consequences of episodes of depression. To achieve these goals, intervention can occur at multiple levels, including individual psychotherapy, family therapy/ education and pharmacological treatment. Treatment should be individualised and based on need, resources and assessment of stressors involved in a particular case. Supportive psychotherapy is an essential component of an individualised treatment plan, independent of whether specific psychotherapies or medication are used.

2.1.1 Supportive Psychotherapy

Supportive psychotherapy will address individual, family, school and social precipitants and consequences of depression. Individually, the child/ adolescent will be assisted in coping with depressed mood. The aim is for the child to spend as much of the day as possible functioning normally, regardless of how they may feel inside. Allowing depressed children to ruminate on their bad feelings continuously does little to improve the situation and, in fact, worsens their depression. Instead, they are encouraged to talk about ways to divert themselves from thinking about their bad feelings. Daily attendance at school and continuing activities is very important, as depressed children's tendency to withdraw from activities and avoid social contact further compounds the depression and hampers recovery.

2.1.2 Other Support

An assessment to evaluate the pre-morbid level of family functioning, marital relationship, impact of illness on the family, family's understanding of the disorder and their attempts to manage it should be conducted at the start of treatment. Education about mood disorders is essential for parents and children. It decreases self-blame and the tendency to blame others. Parents need to know that mood disorders are biological conditions and not personality flaws. Rather than punishment for unacceptable behaviour, the child needs reassurance and support. The family should then assist in the development of a treatment plan, including identifying problem areas for change. Additionally, 30 to 50% of depressed adolescents have a parent who is affectively ill at the time of treatment. Thus, the appropriate identification of parents who need treatment is important in the management of these patients.

The school setting is significant in the treatment process. Often, treatment includes adapting the patient's school setting in order to reduce stress, such as shortening the school day, limiting the amount of school work, developing assignment completion checklists, etc.[51,52] For the learning-disabled child, continuous focus on deficits can lead to worsening mood symptoms. Developing a proactive school environment is essential for these children.

Many children and adolescents with depression have interpersonal problems resulting from social deficits. These deficits compound their depression and often contribute to their feelings of worthlessness, hopelessness and alienation. It is important for therapists, parents and teachers to clarify reality for these patients through role-play, problem-solving techniques, communication and assertiveness training, and conflict resolution.

2.2 Specific Psychotherapies

In addition to supportive psychotherapy and family and school interventions as adjunctive treatments for depression, there is increasing evidence that specific psychotherapies (primarily cognitive, cognitive behavioural and interpersonal therapy) are effective treatments for depression, specifically in adolescents. Although there have been no head-to-head comparisons of depression-specific therapies and medication, available comparative data would suggest equal efficacy. However, the number of adequately trained cognitive and interpersonal therapists is limited. Nonspecific supportive therapy is an essential component to medical management of depression, but has not been shown to be equally effective by itself.[53]

Cognitive therapy, cognitive behavioural therapy and interpersonal therapy are primarily individual treatments, although modifications for adolescents as compared with adults have addressed the necessity of increased involvement of family members.[54] Also, group cognitive behaviour therapy has been extensively studied, and appears to be effective both in depressed and at-risk adolescents.[55-59] Cognitive behavioural therapy is generally time-limited and focused on identifying thought patterns which make the child feel depressed. A recent study by Brent et al.[53] compared cognitive behaviour therapy, systematic-behavioural family therapy, or individual nondirective supportive therapy, and found rates of remission to be 60, 37 and 39%, respectively. Mufson and Fairbanks [60] reported positive results of interpersonal psychotherapy in adolescents with depression both in acute treatment and for 1 year following treatment.

Table I. Factors to consider in determining whether or not to treat depressed children and adolescents with medication

Severity of depression
Other family members' response
Recurrent depression
Not the first episode
Has not responded to psychotherapy
Convenience for family
Presence of psychosocial stressors

2.3 Medication Management

2.3.1 Initial Treatment

The initial decision in medication management is whether to begin a trial of antidepressants. Primarily, decisions about antidepressant use in children and adolescents have been influenced by data from adults.[61] However, increasing evidence is available to make medication decisions from data available specifically in children and adolescents, as well as extrapolating from adult data. Table I lists factors to consider in deciding whether or not to use medication. The clinician must actively involve the patient and family in the decision process.

Assuming that the symptoms of depression are persistent in the depressed child in spite of preliminary psychosocial interventions, then the initial decision is which medication to use as the first line of treatment. There is overwhelming evidence that selective serotonin (5-hydroxy-tryptamine; 5-HT) reuptake inhibitors (SSRIs) are the initial medication choice in this age group. Several well-designed trials of tricyclic antidepressants (TCAs) in children and adolescents have failed to demonstrate effectiveness compared with placebo.[62] Conversely, two recent trials in children and adolescents have shown the effectiveness of fluoxetine[37] and paroxetine (in adolescents).[63] Additionally, adverse effects are substantially less with SSRIs than with TCAs[63] and, of particular relevance in adolescents, they are safer when taken in overdose. Research is currently being conducted in the use of noradrenaline (norepinephrine) and serotonin reuptake inhibitors, such as nefazadone and venlafaxine, in the treatment of children and adolescents with depression. Table II lists approximate dosages for medications in paediatric populations.

The goal of acute treatment is symptom remission, not just symptom improvement. Although no specific data are available in children and adolescents, partial remission increases the risk for relapse in adults. However, remission may take up to 12 weeks.[8]

2.3.2 Treatment-Resistant Depression

Based on adult treatment guidelines from the Texas Medication Algorithm Project (TMAP),[64] failure to respond to an initial SSRI would lead to a trial of an alternative SSRI, followed by an alternative class of antidepressants or augmentation of an SSRI with lithium or buspirone. Table III lists the advantages and disadvantages of switching medications versus augmentation. However, prior to making changes, it is important to reassess the accuracy of the initial diagnosis and the presence of previously unrecognised conditions. The following factors should be considered:

(i) Are there previously unrecognised comorbid diagnoses, such as attention deficit hyperactivity disorder (ADHD), or anxiety, bipolar, substance abuse or eating disorders?

(ii) Are there unrecognised medical conditions?

(iii) Has the patient been compliant with treatment?

(iv) Are there new or additional psycho-social factors affecting treatment?

(v) Is there family dysfunction or psychopathology in family members that require more intensive treatment?

Failure of treatment can also result from adverse effects. It is important to separate the use of additional medication to treat adverse effects from the use of additional medication to augment the initial treatment response. Adverse events seen with SSRIs include insomnia and behavioural activation. Insomnia is a common symptom of depression and also an adverse effect of SSRIs,[63,67] so many clinicians prescribe SSRIs in combination with trazodone or another sedating antidepressant. However, the insomnia frequently improves with continued treatment with the SSRI alone, and often combined treatment is unnecessary.

Table II. Approximate dosages for antidepressants in children

Medication	Paediatric dosage (mg/day)	How supplied (in US)
SSRIs		
Citalopram	10-30	20 and 40mg tablets
Fluoxetine	10-30	10 and 20mg capsules, and concentrate
Fluvoxamine	25-150	50 and 100mg tablets
Paroxetine	10-30	10, 20 and 30mg tablets
Sertraline	25-200	25, 50 and 100mg tablets
Others		
Nefazodone	50-300	100, 150 and 200mg tablets
Venlafaxine	37.5-150	37.5, 75 and 150mg capsules

SSRIs = selective serotonin (5-hydroxytryptamine; 5-HT) reuptake inhibitors.

Table III. Advantages and disadvantages of switching versus augmentation after failure to respond to initial antidepressant medication (modified from Howland & Thase[65] and Thase & Rush[66])

Advantages of switching
Possible different mechanisms of action
Lower risk of drug interaction
Possibly fewer adverse effects
Possibly better adherence to treatment
Possibly less expensive

Disadvantages of switching
Need for discontinuation of initial antidepressant
Lag in response
Possible loss of partial response to prior treatment
Possible loss of drug-drug synergy

A proportion of children treated with antidepressants will manifest a worsening of their behaviour. In some patients this is due to development of manic symptoms. Approximately 3 to 6% of children with severe depression can switch to develop manic symptoms; the rate is probably not different between those treated with SSRIs or with TCAs. Whether the rate of manic switching is higher in children and adolescents than in adults is not clear, but is possible given the early onset and the fact that bipolar disorder often presents initially as depression. For the majority of patients, manic symptoms subside quickly with the discontinuation of the antidepressant.

2.3.3 Continuation Treatment

Substantial information exists that relapse and recurrence (new episode) of depression occur naturalistically in children and adolescents at rates equal to or surpassing the rates in adults. However, no controlled data are available specific to children and adolescents. Therefore, the guideline for how long to treat an episode of depression in children and adolescents following remission is the same as in adults, i.e. 4 to 6 months. However, it is not possible at this time to determine which patients require maintenance treatment, i.e. treatment to prevent new episodes of depression. Patients with severe depression and a history of previous episodes are likely to be treated for a longer period of time than 4 to 6 months but, unlike in adults, it is premature to assume that a certain number of previous episodes would necessarily imply a need for life-long treatment.

3. Conclusion

Diagnosing depressive disorders in children and adolescents requires substantial clinical acumen. Failure to identify these problems will often lead to undertreatment, or less than adequate treatment, of a potentially curable condition. The process of making an appropriate diagnosis includes direct interviewing of the child and primary caretakers, using a semistructured close-ended interview process, and obtaining a detailed systematic family history of mood disorders. The simultaneous presentation of symptoms of other psychiatric, neurological and general medical conditions will often complicate the process.

Primary mood disorders are rarely isolated episodes, and an understanding of the course of illness is essential to appropriate management. Many children and adolescents will have recurrent episodes. Additionally, the ability to identify states that are precursors to major depression would allow the possibility of developing strategies for prevention.

Although it is possible that preliminary indications of treatment efficacy can be extrapolated from studies in adults, there is sufficient difference between adult mood disorders and mood disorders in children and adolescents to require that all treatments be evaluated specifically in this population. There appears to be a consensus that the first-line medication for MDD in an adolescent is an SSRI, primarily because of a putative broader range of action, limited adverse effect profile and relative safety in overdose. However, continued research is needed on the effectiveness of psychotherapy and medication, and the safety of medication, in children and adolescents. Similarly, little is known about how long to continue treatment once it has been shown to be effective. Finally, in treating children and adolescents who have depression it is essential that serious consideration be given to the effects of the psychosocial stressors that may have a role in the child's depression, and to adjust treatment accordingly.

Acknowledgements

This work was supported in part by grants from the National Institutes of Mental Health MH-39188.

References
1. Fleming JE, Offord DR. Epidemiology of childhood depressive disorders: a critical review. J Am Acad Child Adolesc Psychiatry 1990; 29: 571-80
2. Brent DA. Correlates of the medical lethality of suicide attempts in children and adolescents. J Am Acad Child Adolesc Psychiatry 1987; 26: 87-91
3. Pfeffer CR, Klerman GL, Hurt SW, et al. Suicidal children grow up: demographic and clinical risk factors for adolescent suicide attempts. J Am Acad Child Adolesc Psychiatry 1991; 30: 609-16
4. Shaffer D, Fisher P, Dulcan MK, et al. The NIMH diagnostic interview schedule for children version 2.3 (DISC-2.3): description, acceptability, prevalence rates, and performance in the MECA study. Methods for the epidemiology of child and adolescent mental disorders study. J Am Acad Child Adolesc Psychiatry 1996; 35 (7): 865-77
5. Kessler RC, McGonagle KA, Nelson CB, et al. Sex and depression in the national comorbidity survey: II. Cohort effects. J Affect Disord 1994; 30: 15-26
6. Emslie GJ, Weinberg WA, Rush AJ, et al. Depressive symptoms by self report in adolescence: phase I of the development of a questionnaire for depression by self-report. J Child Neurol 1990; 3: 114-21
7. Angold A, Costello EJ, Worthman CM. Puberty and depression: the roles of age, pubertal status and pubertal timing. Psychol Med 1998; 28: 51-61
8. Emslie GJ, Rush AJ, Weinberg WA, et al. Fluoxetine in child and adolescent depression: acute and maintenance treatment. Depress Anxiety 1998; 7: 32-9

9.   American Psychiatric Association: diagnostic and statistical manual of mental disorders. 4th Ed. Washington, DC: American Psychiatric Association, 1994

10. Kaufman J, Birmaher B, Brent D, et al. Schedule for Affective Disorders and Schizophrenia for School-Age Children – Present and Lifetime Version (K-SADS-PL): initial reliability and validity data. J Am Acad Child Adolesc Psychiatry 1997; 36: 980-8

11. Kovacs M. Children's Depression Inventory (CDI). Psychopharmacol Bull 1985; 21: 995-8

12. Weinberg WA, Harper CR, Emslie GJ. Weinberg depression scale for children and adolescents. Austin, Texas: Pro-Ed International Publisher, 1998

13. Kovacs M, Feinberg TL, Crouse-Novak MA. Depressive disorders in childhood: I. A longitudinal prospective study of characteristics and recovery. Arch Gen Psychiatry 1984; 41: 229-37

14. Akiskal HS, Downs J, Jordan P, et al. Affective disorders in referred children and younger siblings of manic-depressives: mode of onset and prospective course. Arch Gen Psychiatry 1985; 42 (10): 996-1003

15. Kovacs M. Presentation and course of major depressive disorder during childhood and later years of the life span. J Am Acad Child Adolesc Psychiatry 1996; 35 (6): 705-15

16. Rao U, Ryan ND, Birmaher B, et al. Unipolar depression in adolescents: clinical outcome in adulthood. J Am Acad Child Adolesc Psychiatry 1995; 34: 566-78

17. Puig-Antich J, Goetz D, Davies M, et al. A controlled family history study of prepubertal major depressive disorder. Arch Gen Psychiatry 1989; 46: 406-18

18. Rutter M, Graham P, Yule W. A neuropsychiatric study in childhood. In: Clinics in developmental medicine, no. 35-36. London: Spastics Society/Heinemann Medical, 1970

19. Cantwell D, Baker L. Academic failures in children with communication disorders. J Am Acad Child Psychiatry 1980; 19: 579-91

20. Robinson RG, Boston JD, Starkstein SE, et al. Comparison of mania and depression after brain injury: causal factors. Am J Psychiatry 1988; 145 (2): 172-8

21. Robinson RG, Starkstein SE. Current research in affective disorders following stroke. J Neuropsychiatry Clin Neurosci 1990; 2: 1-14

22. Starkstein SE, Mayberg HS, Berthier ML, et al. Mania after brain injury: neuroradiological and metabolic findings. Ann Neurol 1990; 27 (6): 652-9

23. Barraclough B. Suicide and epilepsy. In: Reynolds EH, Trimble MR, editors. Epilepsy and psychiatry. Edinburgh: Churchill Livingstone, 1981: 72-6

24. Robertson MM. The organic contribution to depressive illness in patients with epilepsy. J Epilepsy 1989; 2: 189-230

25. Ring HA, Trimble MR. Depression in epilepsy. In: Starkstein SE, Robinson RG, editors. Depression in neurological disease. Baltimore, MD: Johns Hopkins Press, 1993: 63-83

26. Rutter M, Tizard J, Yule W, et al. Research report: Isle of Wight Studies, 1964-1974. Psychol Med 1976; 6: 313-32

27. Ling W, Oftedal G, Weinberg W. Depressive illness in childhood presenting as severe headache. Am J Dis Child 1970; 120: 122-4

28. Weinberg WA, Rutman J, Sullivan L, et al. Depression in children referred to an educational diagnostic center: diagnosis and treatment. J Pediatr 1973; 83: 1065-72

29. Weinberg WA, Rehmet A. Childhood affective disorder and school problems. In: Cantwell DP, Carlson GA, editors. Affective disorders in childhood and adolescence: an update. Jamaica, NY: Spectrum Publications, 1983: 109-28

30. Livingston R. Depressive illness and learning difficulties: research needs and practical implications. J Learn Disabil 1985; 18: 518-20

31. Emslie GJ, Kennard BD, Kowatch RA. Affective disorders in children: diagnosis and management. J Child Neurol 1995; 10 Suppl. 1: S42-S49

32. Brumback RA, Weinberg WA. Pediatric behavioral neurology: an update on the neurological aspects of depression, hyperactivity, and learning disabilities. Neurol Clin 1990; 8 (3): 677-703

33. Brumback RA, Deitz-Schmidt SG, Weinberg WA. Depression in children referred to an educational diagnostic center: diagnosis and treatment and analysis of criteria and literature review. Dis Nerv System 1977; 38: 529-35

34. Biederman J, Farone SV, Keenan K, et al. Evidence of familial association between attention deficit disorder and major affective disorders. Arch Gen Psychiatry 1991; 48: 633-42

35. McCauley E, Myers K, Mitchell J, et al. Depression in young people: initial presentation and clinical course. J Am Acad Child Adolesc Psychiatry 1993; 32 (4): 714-22

36. Strober M, Lampert C, Schmidt S, et al. The course of major depressive disorder in adolescents: I. Recovery and risk of manic switching in a follow-up of psychotic and nonpsychotic subtypes. J Am Acad Child Adolesc Psychiatry 1993; 32 (1): 34-42

37. Emslie GJ, Rush AJ, Weinberg WA, et al. Recurrence of major depressive disorder in hospitalized children and adolescents. J Am Acad Child Adolesc Psychiatry 1997; 36: 785-92

38. Keller MB, Beardslee W, Lavori PW, et al. Course of major depression in non-referred adolescents: a retrospective study. J Affect Disord 1988; 15: 235-43

39. Keller MB, Lavori PW, Beardslee WR, et al. Depression in children and adolescents: new data on 'undertreatment' and a literature review on the efficacy of available treatments. J Affect Disord 1991; 21: 163-71

40. Keller MB, Lavori PW, Mueller TI, et al. Time to recovery, chronicity, and levels of psychopathology in major depression. A 5-year prospective follow-up of 431 subjects. Arch Gen Psychiatry 1992; 49: 809-16

53

41. Coryell W, Akiskal HS, Leon AC, et al. The time course of nonchronic major depressive disorder. Uniformity across episodes and samples. National Institute of Mental Health Collaborative Program on the Psychobiology of Depression – Clinical Studies. Arch Gen Psychiatry 1994; 51: 405-10

42. Asarnow JR, Goldstein MJ, Carlson GA, et al. Childhood-onset depressive disorders: a follow-up study of rates of rehospitalization and out-of-home placement among child psychiatric inpatients. J Affect Disord 1988; 15: 245-53

43. Eastgate J, Gilmour L. Long-term outcome of depressed children: a follow-up study. Dev Med Child Neurol 1984; 26: 68-72

44. Goodyer I, Germany E, Gowrusankur J, et al. Social influences on the course of anxious and depressive disorders in school-age children. Br J Psychiatry 1991; 158: 676-84

45. Poznanski EO, Krahenbuhl V, Zrull JP. Childhood depression. J Am Acad Child Adolesc Psychiatry 1976; 15: 491-501

46. Fleming JE, Boyle MH, Offord DR. The outcome of adolescent depression in the Ontario child health study follow-up. J Am Acad Child Adolesc Psychiatry 1993; 32 (1): 28-33

47. McGee R, Williams S. A longitudinal study of depression in nine-year-old children. J Am Acad Child Adolesc Psychiatry 1988; 27 (3): 342-8

48. Garber J, Kriss MR, Koch M, et al. Recurrent depression in adolescents: a follow-up study. J Am Acad Child Adolesc Psychiatry 1988; 27: 49-54

49. Kovacs M, Feinberg TL, Crouse-Novak MA. Depressive disorders in childhood: II. A longitudinal study of the risk for a subsequent major depression. Arch Gen Psychiatry 1984; 41: 643-9

50. Harrington R, Fudge H, Rutter M, et al. Adult outcomes of childhood and adolescent depression. Arch Gen Psychiatry 1990; 47: 465-73

51. Weinberg WA, Harper CR, Emslie GJ. The effect of depression and learning disabilities on school behavior problems. Direct Clin Psychol 1994; 4: 1-21

52. Weinberg WA, McLean A. A diagnostic approach to developmental specific learning disorders. J Child Neurol 1986; 1 (2): 158-72

53. Brent DA, Holder D, Kolko D, et al. A clinical psychotherapy trial for adolescent depression comparing cognitive, family, and supportive therapy. Arch Gen Psychiatry 1997; 54: 877-85

54. Wilkes TCR, Rush AJ. Case study - adaptations of cognitive therapy for depressed adolescents. J Am Acad Child Adolesc Psychiatry 1988; 27 (3): 381-6

55. Clarke GN, Hawkins W, Murphy M, et al. Targeted prevention of unipolar depressive disorder in an at-risk sample of high school adolescents: a randomized trial of a group cognitive intervention. J Am Acad Child Adolesc Psychiatry 1995; 34: 312-21

56. Reynolds WM, Coats KI. A comparison of cognitive-behavioral therapy and relaxation training for the treatment of depression in adolescents. J Consult Clin Psychol 1986; 54: 653-60

57. Kahn JS, Kehle TJ, Jenson WR, et al. Comparison of cognitive-behavioral, relaxation, and self-modeling interventions for depression among middle-school students. Sch Psychol Rev 1990; 19: 195-210

58. Lewinsohn PM, Clarke GN, Hops H, et al. Cognitive-behavioral treatment for depressed adolescents. Behav Ther 1990; 21: 385-401

59. Lewinsohn PM, Clarke GN, Rhode P, et al. A course in coping: a cognitive-behavioral approach to the treatment of adolescent depression. In: Hibb ED, Jensen PS, editors. Psychosocial treatments for children and adolescent disorders: empirically based strategies for clinical practice. Washington, DC: American Psychiatric Association Press, 1996: 109-35

60. Mufson L, Fairbanks J. Interpersonal psychotherapy for depressed adolescents: a one-year naturalistic follow-up study. J Am Acad Child Adolesc Psychiatry 1995; 35: 1145-55

61. Depression Guideline Panel. Depression in primary care: detection and diagnosis. Clinical practice guideline. Vol. 1 (5). Rockville, MD: US Department of Health and Human Services, Public Health Service, Agency for Health Care Policy and Research. AHCPR Publication No. 93-0550, 1993

62. Hazell P, O'Connell D, Heathcote D, et al. Efficacy of tricyclic drugs in treating child and adolescent depression: a meta-analysis. BMJ 1995; 310: 897-901

63. Wagner KD, Birmaher B, Carlson G, et al. Safety of paroxetine and imipramine in the treatment of adolescent depression. Presented at the New Clinical Drug Evaluation Unit Program (NCDEW), 38th Annual Meeting. 1998; Boca Raton, FL

64. Gilbert DA, Altshuler KZ, Rago WV, et al. Texas medication algorithm project: definitions, rationale, and methods to develop medication algorithms. J Clin Psychiatry 1998; 59: 345-51

65. Howland RH, Thase ME. Switching strategies for the treatment of unipolar major depression. Mod Probl Pharmacopsychiatry 1997; 25: 56-65

66. Thase ME, Rush AJ. When at first you don't succeed: sequential strategies for antidepressant nonresponders. J Clin Psychiatry 1997; 58 Suppl.: 23-9

67. Pierce LY, Emslie GJ. Fluoxetine side effects [abstract]. Scientific proceedings of the 42nd Annual Meeting of the American Academy of Child and Adolescent Psychiatry. New Orleans, Oct 1995

Correspondence: Dr *Graham J. Emslie*, The University of Texas Southwestern Medical Center, 5323 Harry Hines Boulevard, Dallas, TX 75235-8897, USA.

Schizophrenic Psychoses in Childhood and Adolescence
A Guide to Diagnosis and Drug Choice

Helmut Remschmidt, Eberhard Schulz and *Beate Herpertz-Dahlmann*

Department of Child and Adolescent Psychiatry, Philipps University, Marburg, Germany

1. Epidemiology

Psychoses in childhood that meet the DSM-IV[1] criteria for schizophrenia are rare, with a prevalence of only 0.19 per 10 000 in children aged 2 to 12 years.[2] In childhood-onset schizophrenia, boys predominate, with a reported gender ratio of about 2 to 2.5 : 1.[3-5] Furthermore, boys appear to have an earlier onset of schizophrenic symptoms and poorer premorbid histories than girls.[5,6]

2. Classification

There is a growing body of evidence demonstrating that age and developmental stage at onset are the most important factors for the subgrouping and classification of childhood psychoses.[3,7-16] Based on this approach, at least four groups of psychoses in childhood and adolescence can be differentiated (table I).[17]

The first group of psychoses comprises various psychotic syndromes characterised by a gradual onset, chronic course and manifestation before the third year of life. None of the psychotic syndromes within this group, with the exception of early infantile catatonia,[21] has any relationship to adult-onset schizophrenia. The second group embraces the psychotic states, most of them with an acute onset between the third and fifth years of life and featuring regressive behaviour of various kinds. Their relationship to schizophrenia is also questionable, again with the probable exception of early infantile catatonia. The third group of psychoses is characterised by an age at onset between late childhood and prepuberty, a fluctuating or sub-acute course and a clear relationship to schizophrenia of adolescence and adulthood. This applies especially to prepubertal schizophrenia. The fourth group comprises adolescent schizophrenia with a manifestation of the psychosis during puberty and adolescence. This type of the disorder is very clearly related to schizophrenia of adulthood.

Some authors[16] proposed to distinguish between early-onset schizophrenia, defined as beginning in childhood or adolescence (i.e. before age 16 or 17 years), and very early-onset schizophrenia, with an onset before 13 years of age. The argument in favour of using the latter definition is that it is more precise than the term 'prepubertal', because puberty may vary in relation to age, and most studies that have used the term prepubertal schizophrenia have not taken the pubertal stages into consideration.

In any respect, while considering age and developmental stages for the classification of

Table I. Psychotic syndromes that can occur in childhood and adolescence, and their relationship to schizophrenia[14]

Clinical syndrome	Age at onset	Course	Relationship to schizophrenia
Group I Kanner autism[18] Pseudodefective psychosis[19,20]	Before third year of life	Chronic	None
Early infantile catatonia[21]	Possibly before third year of life		Likely
Group II	Between third and fifth years of life	Acute: regressive behaviour	Questionable
Dementia infantilis[22] Dementia praecocissima[23] Pseudoneurotic schizophrenia[19,20] Acute-onset type[24] Symbiotic psychosis[25,26] Asperger syndrome[27,28]			
Early infantile catatonia[21]	Usually within the first 6 years of life		Likely
Group III	Late childhood and prepuberty	Fluctuating, subacute	Related to schizophrenia of adolescence and adulthood
Psychoses (late-onset psychoses)[10-13] Pseudopsychopathic schizophrenia[20] Prepubertal schizophrenia[29]	Prepuberty		Clear
Group IV Adolescent schizophrenia[30]	Puberty and adolescence		Clear

childhood psychoses, recently obtained research data confirmed the notion of Kanner,[18,31] who had subdivided psychoses in childhood into three groups: (i) early infantile autism; (ii) childhood schizophrenia; and (iii) disintegrative psychoses of childhood. The latter comprises disorders such as Heller's infantile dementia and psychoses related to different kinds of brain damage.[22,32] These distinctions have influenced multiaxial classification systems[33] based on ICD-9[34] and ICD-10,[35] and DSM-III,[36] DSM-III-R[37] and DSM-IV, which differentiate between early infantile autism, schizophrenia and (early childhood) dementia.

3. Diagnosis

Based on studies that classified children with psychoses according to age at onset and the specific developmental factors present, it is suggested that schizophrenia and early-onset developmental disorders may be unrelated and constitute distinct disorders.[3,38-40] In this regard, it is argued that childhood schizophrenia is a variant of, and differing only quantitatively from, the manifestation of the disorder in adulthood.[41] Following these lines of argument, the three most recent editions of DSM eliminated childhood schizophrenia as a separate disorder, and children received the diagnosis of schizophrenia if they met the adult criteria.

Most cases of early-onset and adolescent schizophrenia are characterised by an insidious onset,[5,42] with a long history of precursors of both positive and negative symptoms.[42,43] In the early manifestations of schizophrenia, premorbid characteristics with introversive symptoms (e.g. mutism, social isolation, general anxieties, obsessive-compulsive symptoms) predominate over extraversive behavioural patterns (e.g. hyperactivity, aggression, school refusal). In addition to the psychopathological symptoms, childhood schizophrenia appears to be linked to disabilities including attentional and information processing impairments as well as delays in speech and motor development.[6,10,39,42,44-48]

With respect to developmental aspects, King[39] has pointed to some of the difficulties that arise from the strict application of adult criteria for diagnosing schizophrenia in childhood (in this case, DSM-III-R criteria, but the problems also occur with DSM-IV criteria):

Table II. Distribution of psychotic symptoms according to studies of childhood-onset schizophrenia[49]

Parameter	Kolvin et al.[52]	Russell et al.[4]	Green et al.[5]
No. of patients	33	35	38
Male : female ratio	24 : 9	24 : 11	26 : 12
Mean age at diagnosis	11.1	9.5	9.6
(range) [years]	(5-15)	(4.8-13.3)	(5.7-11.11)
Psychotic symptoms (%)			
Auditory hallucinations	82	80	84.2
Visual hallucinations	30	37	47.4
Delusions	58	63	55.3
Thought disorder	60	40	100

- most children with schizophrenia manifest nonspecific difficulties and vulnerabilities as early as the first or second year of life;
- pathognomonic signs of schizophrenia are rarely seen before the age of 5 or 6 years;
- the presence or absence of hallucinations, delusions and formal thought disorder may be difficult to ascertain in very young and linguistically impaired children;
- in young children it can be difficult to distinguish bizarre ideas, preoccupations, phobias or obsessions from delusions.

Regardless of these difficulties, studies on childhood psychoses were able to show that most of the children with schizophrenia met the DSM-III- R criteria, and that schizophrenia can be diagnosed in children using the same criteria as those used for adults.[3-5,10,40,49-53]

The major recent studies of childhood-onset schizophrenia demonstrate that psychotic symptoms show a typical distribution (see table II).[49] In samples of children selected to meet the criteria for schizophrenia as outlined in DSM-III or DSM-III-R, auditory hallucinations occurred in about 80%, visual hallucinations in 30 to 47%, and tactile and haptic hallucinations in only a few cases. Delusions are reported in 55 to 63% of cases. Depending on the assessment criteria, thought disorder was found in 40 to 100% of children with schizophrenia, and about 70% of the childhood cases were characterised by flat or inappropriate affect.[39,49] According to the classification schemes, the paranoid-hallucinatory and the undifferentiated type were the predominant clinical diagnostic subtypes in cases of early-onset schizophrenia. Catatonic behaviour was reported only infrequently.[39,42,43,54]

3.1 Differential Diagnosis

With respect to differential diagnosis, it is important to consider that developmental factors influence the form and content of psychotic symptoms.[55] In this regard, childhood hallucinations require very careful examination and, at the minium, the following information should be obtained:[56]

- the sensory type of the hallucinations;
- a complete description of the symptoms – including intermittent or continuous, infrequent or common, ill-defined or clear, simple or complex, fragmented or organised;
- whether the child can appreciate the pathological nature of the hallucinations;
- occurrence of imagery and pseudo-hallucinations;
- the state of consciousness;
- the presence of associated disease – functional or organic;
- psychological content and function.

In addition, a differential diagnosis has to take into account normal phenomena of childhood, such as imaginary companions and night terrors.[56-58]

Only by differential diagnosis based on physical, neurological (in some cases completed by neuroimaging and laboratory data) and neuropsychological evaluation and a careful examination of the child's personality structure, as well as the form and content of the symptoms, can one arrive at the diagnosis of hallucinations, delusions and thought disorders. From a developmental psychopathological point of view, it becomes evident that hallucinations are not pathognomonic of childhood schizophrenia. They also occur in acute anxiety states, adjustment reactions as transient situational responses, deprived children with developing personality disorders of various types, and mentally retarded children. In childhood, isolated hallucinations are usually associated with depressive states, anxiety and social difficulties.[39,51,55,56,59-61] Table III outlines those disorders that have to be differentiated from childhood schizophrenia.

4. Treatment Strategies: Overview

Five different measures have been proven to be relevant to the treatment of psychoses in children and adolescents:[17,30,42,63] (i) pharmacological treatment of acute psychotic states; (ii) pharmacological prevention of relapses; (iii) psychotherapeutic measures; (iv) family-oriented measures; and (v) specific measures of rehabilitation. It should be emphasised that pharmacotherapy has to be part of a comprehensive treatment plan, which also includes psychotherapeutic and family-oriented interventions. An important therapeutic aim is to provide clear, adequate information about the disorder, related problems, and the risks and benefits of drug treatment strategies to the patient and his/her parents.

In psychotic states, psychotherapeutic measures should have a predominantly supportive role rather than one that is conflict-revealing. Similar to the treatment of schizophrenic psychoses in adulthood, the young patient has to learn how to cope with different kinds of stress in a way that can prevent relapses. Training programmes on the basic cognitive deficits have been proved to be effective,[64,65] and they are of special relevance for the outcome of the disorder.

Attention must be paid to the secondary sequelae of the psychotic process and their effects on the child and his/her family. In this regard, it is self-evident that the families of children with psychosis have to be included in the plan and concept of therapy. However, empirical research has shown that the ambitious family therapy concepts that have been propagated during the last two decades have not provided the benefits that were hoped for.[66,67] Empirically based research has failed to show that families labelled as typically 'psychotic' or 'schizophrenogenic' really exist.[67] However, studies using the concept of expressed emotions demonstrated that emotional factors within the family play an important role in the prevention or provocation of relapses within the course of the disorder.[67,68] Therefore, in every case of childhood psychosis, one has to decide on the extent to which the family should be integrated

Table III. Disorders that have to be considered in making a differential diagnosis of childhood schizophrenia[39,42,43,51,62]

Adjustment reactions
Affective disorders
Autism and pervasive developmental disorder
Brain damage
Drug-induced psychotic states
Intoxications
Metabolic and hormonal disturbances
Neurotic disorders
Seizure disorders
Schizotypal and borderline personality disorders
Viral infections

Table IV. Commonly used antipsychotics, with their relative potency and dosage range

Class	Drug	Chlorpromazine equivalents (in mg)	Daily dose (mg) [mg/kg/day] children	adolescents
Phenothiazines				
aliphatic	Chlorpromazine	100	10-200 [0.5-3.0]	50-600
piperidine	Thioridazine	97	10-200 [0.5-3.0]	50-600
piperizine	Trifluoperazine	2.8	2-20	Not studied
Butyrophenones	Haloperidol	1.6	0.25-6.0	1.0-16
Thioxanthenes	Thiothixene	8.8	1.0-6.0 [0.1-2.0]	5.0-45
Dihydroindolones	Molindone	6.0	1.0-155 [0.1-2.0]	75-255
Dibenzoxazepines	Loxapine	17.4	Not studied	25-200
Diphenylbutylpiperidine	Pimozide	0.3-0.5	1-6 [≤ 0.3]	1-9 [≤ 0.3]
Dibenzodiazepines	Clozapine	50	Not studied	100-700

into the therapeutic process. This depends on the patient, the course of the disorder, the structure and stability of the family, and the experience of the therapist.

5. Pharmacological Treatment

The pharmacological treatment of children and adolescents with schizophrenia is characterised by a paucity of empirical studies evaluating the efficacy and safety of antipsychotic drugs. Despite this lack of data, clinical trials in adolescents with schizophrenia indicate that antipsychotic medication can be considered to be a specific and effective treatment strategy. Table IV lists some of the antipsychotics that are commonly used in children and adolescents, with relative potencies and recommended dosage ranges.[69]

5.1 Drug Choice

5.1.1 Typical Antipsychotics
To the best of our knowledge, only three double-blind, placebo-controlled studies of the effect of typical antipsychotics in children or adolescents have been published.[70-72] Furthermore, only one of these studies involved children who fulfilled the DSM-III-R criteria for schizophrenia.[70]

The latter study is still ongoing.[53,70] It is a 10-week crossover study involving 16 children with DSM-III-R–defined schizophrenia who were a mean age of 8.9 years (range 5.5 to 11.8 years) at the start of treatment. After a 2-week placebo baseline period, patients who continued to show active schizophrenic symptoms are assigned randomly to one of two 8-week treatment sequences: (i) haloperidol for 4 weeks followed by placebo for 4 weeks; or (ii) placebo for 4 weeks followed by haloperidol for 4 weeks. All 16 patients improved while receiving haloperidol, and continued receiving haloperidol after the study. The mean optimal dosage for haloperidol was 1.92 mg/day, or 0.057 mg/kg/day (range: 0.5 to 3.5 mg/day, or 0.02 to 0.12 mg/kg/day). Significant treatment effects for active drug were found using the Clinical Global Impression (CGI) Severity of Illness scale,[73] the CGI Global Improvement scale, the Brief Psychiatric Rating Scale for Children Total Pathology score,[74] and for four of eight selected items on the Children's Psychiatric Rating Scale,[75] including ideas of reference, persecutory, other thinking disorders and hallucinations.

In acute states of schizophrenia (i.e. patients with hallucinations, delusions and excitement), butyrophenones (especially haloperidol) and phenothiazines have been very useful. In patients

Topics in Paediatric Psychiatry

with a more chronic course of schizophrenia, less potent antipsychotics such as thioridazine have been useful. A combination of these substances with levomepromazine and chlorprothixene has been effective in cases of extreme excitement and aggression.[42]

5.1.2 Atypical Antipsychotics

Clozapine

Clozapine has been described as an atypical antipsychotic with greater affinity for dopamine D_1 receptors and lesser affinity for D_2 receptors compared with typical agents, along with high affinities for D_4, serotonin 5-HT_1 and 5-HT_2, α_1 adrenergic, muscarinic and histamine H_1 receptors.[76-79] Because of this atypical profile, clozapine is of considerable importance in the management of treatment-refractory schizophrenia.

Siefen and Remschmidt[80] conducted a retrospective study of 21 inpatients, 12 of whom were below 18 years old (mean age 18.1 years). Clozapine was offered to patients who had shown inadequate clinical response to other antipsychotic medications (for whom there was concern that the psychotic symptoms were becoming chronic) or who had extensive extrapyramidal adverse effects during treatment with typical drugs. Clozapine was administered, over a mean of 133 days, at a mean maximum dosage of 450 mg/day (range 225 to 800 mg/day) and a mean maintenance dosage of 363 mg/day (range 150 to 800 mg/day). The mean time period between the onset of first symptoms and current treatment was 18.6 months. These patients had had a mean of 2.4 prior inpatient hospitalisations, had previously been prescribed a mean of 2.8 different antipsychotic medications, and had shown inadequate therapeutic responses or problematic adverse effects to these drugs.

After treatment with clozapine, marked or complete improvement was observed in most symptoms in 52% (11 of 21) of patients, and at least some degree of improvement occurred in an additional 29% (6 of 21). Four patients did not respond to clozapine and showed no behavioural changes. In general, during treatment with clozapine, the positive symptoms of schizophrenia showed more clinical improvement than the negative symptoms.

In a second and independent study, adolescents with schizophrenia were administered clozapine in open clinical trials.[81] The 36 adolescents (19 males and 17 females) fulfilled DSM-III-R criteria for schizophrenia, and 61% (n = 22) were already in a chronic state of the disorder. The age at the first manifestation of schizophrenia was 14.9 ± 3.7 years; therefore, the time interval from first manifestation of the disorder to the index hospitalisation was a mean of 3.3 years. Thus, clozapine was administered to these individuals after a mean duration of symptomatic schizophrenia of 3.3 years.

The indication for clozapine treatment was a result of at least one of the following three pretreatment conditions: (i) nonresponse to treatment with at least two conventional antipsychotics, typically haloperidol and fluphenazine; (ii) symptom deterioration during prior treatment with typical antipsychotics; and (iii) significant adverse effects during treatment with conventional antipsychotics. During inpatient treatment, the mean dosage of clozapine was 330 mg/day (range 50 to 800 mg/day). The mean duration of these open clinical trials was 154 days (± 93 days).

During clozapine treatment, 11% of patients were rated as showing a complete remission of symptoms (4 of 36), and 75% (27 of 36) were found to have a clinical improvement in symptoms. The rate of improvement of positive symptoms was about 65%. Symptoms that appeared particularly responsive to clozapine were delusions, hallucinations, positive thought disorder symptoms, excitement and attention. With respect to negative symptoms, clozapine was partially effective for symptoms of anergy, mute behaviour, bizarre behaviour and thought blocking. The majority of these patients became able to participate in a comprehensive rehabilitation programme. Only 8% of the individuals (3 of 36) did not show any therapeutic response to clozapine.

In 17% of adolescents (6 of 36), clozapine treatment had to be interrupted because of adverse effects. One patient developed stupor and a worsening of symptoms following 2 weeks of a combination of clozapine (100 mg/day) with carbamazepine (400 mg/day). In 2 patients, the appearance of leucopenia (2900 and 2500 leucocytes/μl) without agranulocytosis led to discontinuation of clozapine. Two patients demonstrated hypertension, tachycardia and electrocardiogram (ECG) abnormalities. One adolescent showed marked elevations of liver transaminases, to levels that were 10-fold above the normal range, without clinical or other laboratory signs of hepatitis.

In an open trial in 11 adolescents with childhood-onset schizophrenia, administration of clozapine was associated with a marked improvement in more than half of the study group.[82] Additional and promising results with clozapine in young schizophrenic patients who were unresponsive to conventional antipsychotics came from a series of case studies and open clinical trials.[83-91]

At present, only limited data are available regarding the appropriate plasma concentrations of clozapine and the response–adverse effects relationships in early-onset schizophrenia. The data so far available are derived from 2 groups of investigators who studied serum or plasma concentrations of clozapine and its major metabolites (*N*-demethyl-clozapine and clozapine *N*-oxide) in samples from adolescents with early-onset schizophrenia.[92,93] The results can be summarised as follows:

(i) In a 1-year follow-up study, 16 adolescent patients received intraindividually fixed doses of clozapine. The individual mean serum concentrations of clozapine and its metabolites from 6 consecutive measurements were calculated for a given fixed dosage of the drug (range 75 to 600 mg/day). Data analysis revealed a strong linear correlation between clozapine dosage and the measured serum concentrations of the drug and its 2 major metabolites.[93]

(ii) Despite this linear relationship, up to 22-fold interindividual differences and a marked intraindividual variability of the measured drug concentrations during follow-up could be observed.[93]

(iii) During maintenance therapy, a trend toward lower scores of positive and negative symptoms in patients exhibiting serum clozapine concentrations of greater than 350 μg/L was found.[93]

(iv) Results obtained in a study sample of 11 adolescents with early-onset schizophrenia revealed that plasma concentrations of clozapine versus clinical benefit exhibited a consistent linear relationship among patients.[92] In this study, dosages were increased on an individual basis to a mean 6-week dosage of 5.99 ± 2.6 mg/kg/day.

Data obtained from an ongoing prospective clinical trial of adolescents with schizophrenia reveal a linear correlation between serum clozapine concentration and adverse effects (Dotes Scale).[93] According to these preliminary findings, patients exhibiting serum concentrations greater than 250 μg/L were at a greater risk of developing adverse effects due to clozapine. The data so far available are limited by small study samples and do not yet allow us to define a therapeutic window or a serum concentration–dosage–adverse effects relationship.

Because of the dose-related increase in the incidence of seizure activity with clozapine, the dose should be increased cautiously, weighing benefit against adverse effects.

Risperidone

In addition to clozapine, risperidone holds promise as an effective atypical antipsychotic in the treatment of schizophrenia.

Risperidone is an antipsychotic agent chemically classified as a benzisoxazole derivative, which has potent $5-HT_2$ and D_2 receptor blocking properties. Data derived from the treatment of adult schizophrenic patients demonstrate that risperidone is an effective atypical antipsychotic, which has beneficial effects on both the negative and the positive symptoms of schizophrenia and is associated with a low incidence of extrapyramidal adverse effects at lower doses.[94] To date, with the exception of single case reports,[95-98] no studies using risperidone in well characterised treatment-refractory children and adolescents with schizophrenia are available.

For further research, comparisons of risperidone and clozapine would be of particular interest.

5.2 Nonresponse

Despite the efficacy of conventional antipsychotics as short term and maintenance treatment of schizophrenia, a high proportion (about 30 to 40%) of patients with early-onset and adolescent schizophrenia are initial nonresponders to typical antipsychotics.[43]

Nonresponse to typical antipsychotics needs careful evaluation of the underlying causes. The most common cause of nonresponse is either incorrect dosage or inadequate duration of treatment (a trial of at least 4 to 6 weeks is recommended to assess the efficacy of an antipsychotic). Noncompliance or pharmacokinetic, pharmacodynamic and pharmacogenetic abnormalities may also be responsible for a lack of response. If these are indicated, serum drug concentration monitoring should be undertaken. This procedure can be considered a useful tool in antipsychotic drug research and in the pharmacological management of early-onset and adolescent schizophrenia.

Before declaring a patient a nonresponder, trials of at least two different typical antipsychotics should be tried, with a selection of antipsychotics from different chemical classes, using adequate dosages.[42,99] If nonresponse can be confirmed, a trial of the atypical antipsychotic clozapine can be considered (see section 5.1.2), if strict guidelines for clinical management are followed. Another option is the use of risperidone. With respect to children and adolescents, no adjunctive agent (lithium, carbamazepine, antidepressants, etc.) has been demonstrated to be markedly effective for the treatment of nonresponders to conventional antipsychotic drugs.

Depot preparations have not been studied in children, and may have inherent risks, as long term exposure to antipsychotics increases the likelihood of adverse effects (see section 6).[69] Therefore, depot antipsychotics should only be considered in adolescents with schizophrenia when compliance with medication is a problem and when there is a poor oral absorption or a strong first-pass effect (i.e. the drug is metabolised by the liver before reaching the brain).[69,99]

5.3 Adverse Effects

Data derived from open clinical trials and retrospective studies suggest that children and adolescents may be more prone to the adverse effects of (and less responsive to) typical antipsychotics than adults.[100-102] Treatment with typical antipsychotics is often discontinued because of severe adverse effects, worsening and deterioration of symptoms (e.g. cognitive impairments, increase in negative symptomatology) or a lack of response.[42,83] The most common adverse effects and reactions that occur after short term treatment with typical antipsychotics in children and adolescents are summarised in table V.[103]

In addition to the short term adverse effects, reported rates of dyskinesias and antipsychotic-induced tardive dyskinesias in children and adolescents vary from 8 to 51%.[104-106] Once antipsychotic treatment has begun, it is recommended to perform assessments for dyskinesias every 3 to 6 months.[99] For a diagnosis of tardive dyskinesias, the following prerequisites must be met:[107,108]

- a minimum of 3 months of cumulative antipsychotic exposure;
- the presence of at least 'moderate' abnormal involuntary movements in one or more body areas (face, lips, jaw, tongue, upper extremities, lower extremities, trunk) and at least 'mild' movements in two or more body areas;
- ratings should be performed using standardised procedures and instruments, such as the Abnormal Involuntary Movement Scale;[73]

Table V. Short term adverse effects of and reactions to typical antipsychotics

Acute dystonia
Affective blunting
Akathisia
Anticholinergic symptoms
Cardiac arrhythmias
Cognitive dulling
Extrapyramidal symptoms
Sedation

Table VI. Disorders that have to be considered in making a differential diagnosis of tardive dyskinesia

Idiopathic dyskinesias
Stereotypies associated with schizophrenia or autism
Blepharospasm-oromandibular dystonia syndrome
Oral dyskinesias secondary to dentures or dental conditions
Idiopathic torsion dystonia
Gilles de la Tourette's disorder and simple tics

Hereditary and systemic illness associated with dyskinesias
Huntington's disease
Sydenham's chorea
Wilson's disease
Encephalitis
Hyperthyroidism
Hypoparathyroidism
Systemic lupus erythematosus
Schönlein-Henoch purpura

- lack of other conditions that might produce abnormal movements (table VI gives on overview of the differential diagnosis of tardive dyskinesia).[103,109]

The prophylactic use of antiparkinsonian drugs to prevent extrapyramidal adverse effects is still a controversial issue. For practical purposes, antiparkinsonian drugs can be considered: (i) in patients who are at high risk of developing extrapyramidal adverse effects (e.g. administered high potency antipsychotics); (ii) when treating new patients; or (iii) in patients in whom there is a risk of impaired compliance due to dystonic adverse effects.

Acute dystonic reactions respond rapidly to anticholinergic and antiparkinsonian drugs, such as diphenhydramine 25 to 50mg orally or intramuscularly, or benzatropine 1 to 2mg intramuscularly. The long term use of antiparkinsonian drugs cannot be recommended for several reasons, including the fact that anticholinergics may aggravate psychotic symptoms and may lower the serum concentrations of antipsychotics.[110]

One of the main advantages of clozapine over traditional antipsychotic medications is that tardive dyskinesias have not yet been observed, and extrapyramidal adverse effects do not occur or, at least, are much less common than with typical antipsychotics. However, clozapine has significant adverse effects of its own, including the induction of agranulocytosis (in approximately 2% of patients) and seizures. As a result, white blood cell counts (at weekly intervals for at least the first 18 weeks of treatment and thereafter at least monthly in European countries, and weekly throughout treatment in the US, in addition to differential cell counts) and EEGs must be monitored. In addition, the data so far available support the need for careful clinical monitoring of a wide range of possible adverse effects of the drug.

6. Treatment Guidelines

Prior to the administration of antipsychotic medication the following issues should be considered:

1. Informed consent – the treatment plan and informed consent for the use of antipsychotic medication should be discussed and, depending on the age of the patient, be signed by the patient and his/her parents.

2. The minimum baseline assessments prior to the initiation of antipsychotics involve careful clinical examinations, a complete medical history (including inquiry for a history of seizures and liver and cardiac diseases), assessment of bodyweight, height, blood pressure and pulse rate, monitoring of EEG and ECG, and laboratory investigations including complete blood count with differential cell counts, and liver function tests.

3. In patients with a history of hypersensitivity to antipsychotics, agranulocytosis associated with antipsychotics, or neuroleptic malignant syndrome added caution is warranted.

A trial of least 4 to 6 weeks is necessary to assess the efficacy of any antipsychotic. There is no evidence to suggest that any one of the typical antipsychotics is superior to another in the treatment of early-onset and adolescent schizophrenia.[69,99] If no clinical improvement is apparent after an initial 4- to 6-week trial, or if severe adverse effects necessitate a cessation of medication, a trial of an alternative typical antipsychotic from a different chemical class should be undertaken. Because of the potential risks of developing tardive dyskinesia and other adverse effects, assessment strategies for prevention and early detection are mandatory (see section 5.3).

In cases of well defined nonresponse to at least two conventional antipsychotics administered at an adequate dosage (see table IV), a trial of the atypical antipsychotic clozapine can be considered, if strict guidelines for clinical management are followed (see section 5.3).

7. Conclusions

The treatment of childhood schizophrenia involves the use of antipsychotic medication as an essential part of a comprehensive treatment plan. This plan should also include social skills training, family therapy and supportive psychotherapy. These measures are cornerstones for rehabilitation and relapse prevention in early-onset schizophrenia.

Data derived from clinical trials of clozapine in adolescents with early-onset schizophrenia demonstrate that this atypical antipsychotic is a possible therapeutic intervention for young patients with schizophrenia who are resistant to conventional treatment strategies. Additional research is needed to further investigate whether clozapine also has beneficial effects in very early-onset schizophrenia in childhood.

References

1. American Psychiatric Association. Diagnostic and statistical manual of mental disorders. 4th ed. Washington, DC: American Psychiatric Association, 1994
2. Burd L, Kerbeshian J. A North Dakota prevalence study of schizophrenia presenting in childhood. J Am Acad Child Adolesc Psychiatry 1987; 26: 347-50
3. Volkmar FR, Cohen DJ, Hoshino Y, et al. Phenomenology and classification of the childhood psychoses. Psychol Med 1988; 18: 191-201
4. Russell AT, Bott L, Sammons C. The phenomenology of schizophrenia occurring in childhood. J Am Acad Child Adolesc Psychiatry 1989; 28 (3): 399-407
5. Green WH, Padron-Gayol M, Hardesty AS, et al. Schizophrenia with childhood onset: a phenomenological study of 38 cases. J Am Acad Child Adolesc Psychiatry 1992; 31: 968-76
6. Watkins JM, Asarnow RF, Tangua P. Symptom development in childhood onset schizophrenia. J Child Psychol Psychiatry 1988; 29: 865-78
7. Anthony EJ. An experimental approach to the psychopathology of childhood autism. Br J Med Psychol 1958; 31: 211-25
8. Anthony EJ. Low-grade psychosis in childhood. In: Richards BW, editor. Proceedings of the London Conference on Scientific Study of Mental Deficiency, vol 2. Dagenham, Essex: May and Baker, 1962: 398-410
9. Bettes BA, Walker E. Positive and negative symptoms in psychotic and other psychiatrically disturbed children. J Child Psychol Psychiatry 1987; 28: 555-68
10. Kolvin I, Ounsted C, Humphrey M, et al. Studies in the childhood psychoses: II. The phenomenology of childhood psychoses. Br J Psychiatry 1971; 118: 385-95
11. Kolvin I, Ounsted C, Richardson LM, et al. Studies in the childhood psychoses: III. The family and social background in childhood psychoses. Br J Psychiatry 1971; 118: 396-402
12. Kolvin I, Garside RF, Kidd JSH. Studies in the childhood psychoses: IV. Parental personality and attitude and childhood psychoses. Br J Psychiatry 1971; 118: 403-6
13. Kolvin I, Ounsted C, Roth M. Studies in the childhood psychoses: V. Cerebral dysfunction and childhood psychoses. Br J Psychiatry 1971; 118: 407-17
14. Remschmidt H. Schizophrene Psychosen im Jugendalter. In: Kisker KP, Lauter H, Meyer J-E, et al., editors. Kinder- und Jugendpsychiatrie. Psychiatrie der Gegenwart, 3rd ed., vol 7. Berlin: Springer-Verlag, 1988: 90-117
15. Werry JS, McClellan JM. Predicting outcome in child and adolescent (early onset) schizophrenia and bipolar disorder. J Am Acad Child Adolesc Psychiatry 1992; 31 (1): 147-50
16. Werry JS. Child and adolescent (early onset) schizophrenia: a review in light of DSM-III-R. J Autism Dev Disord 1992; 22: 601-24
17. Remschmidt H. Schizophrenic psychoses in children and adolescents. Triangle 1993; 32 (1): 15-24
18. Kanner L. Autistic disturbances of affective contact. Nerv Child 1943; 2: 217-50
19. Bender L. Childhood schizophrenia: clinical study of one hundred schizophrenic children. Am J Orthopsychiatry 1947; 17: 40-56
20. Bender L. The concept of pseudopsychopathic schizophrenia in adolescence. Am J Orthopsychiatry 1959; 29: 491-509
21. Leonhard K. Aufteilung der Endogenen Psychosen und ihre differenzierte Ätiologie. 6th ed. Berlin: Akademie Verlag, 1986
22. Heller T. Über Dementia Infantilis. Zeitschrift zur Erforschung und Behandlung Jugendlichen Schwachsinns 1908; 2: 17
23. De Sanctis S. Dementia Praecocissima Catatonica. Folia Neurobiologica 1908; 2: 9
24. Despert JL. Schizophrenia in children. Psychiatr Q 1938; 12: 366-71
25. Mahler MS. On child psychosis and schizophrenia: autistic and symbiotic infantile psychosis. Psychoanal Study Child 1952; 7: 286-305
26. Mahler MS, Ross JR, De Fried Z. Clinical studies in benignant and malignant cases of childhood psychosis (schizophrenic-like). Am J Orthopsychiatry 1949; 19: 295-304
27. Asperger H. Die 'Autistischen Psychopathen' im Kindesalter. Arch Psychiatr Nervenkrank 1944; 117: 76-136
28. Asperger H. Zur Differentialdiagnose des Kindlichen Autismus. Acta Paedopsychiatr 1968; 35: 136-45
29. Stutte H. Psychosen des Kindesalters. In: Opitz H, Schmid F, editors. Handbuch der Kinderheilkunde, vol 8, part 1. Berlin: Springer-Verlag, 1969: 908-37
30. Remschmidt H. Childhood and adolescent schizophrenia. Curr Opin Psychiatry 1993; 6: 470-9
31. Kanner L. Child psychiatry. 3rd ed. Oxford: Blackwell, 1957
32. Stutte H, Harbauer H. Die Nosologie der Dementia infantilis (Heller). Jahrb Jugendpsychiat Grenzgeb 1965; 4: 206-24
33. Rutter ML, Shaffer D, Sturge C. A guide to a multi-axial classification scheme for psychiatric disorders in childhood and adolescence. London: Frowde, 1975
34. World Health Organization. International statistical classification of diseases and related health problems. 9th ed., vol 1. Geneva: World Health Organization, 1977
35. World Health Organization. International statistical classification of diseases and related health problems. 10th ed., vol 1. Geneva: World Health Organization, 1991
36. American Psychiatric Association. Diagnostic and statistical manual of mental disorders. 3rd ed. Washington, DC: American Psychiatric Association, 1980
37. American Psychiatric Association. Diagnostic and statistical manual of mental disorders. 3rd rev ed. Washington, DC: American Psychiatric Association, 1987
38. Kolvin I. Studies in the childhood psychoses: I. Diagnostic criteria and classification. Br J Psychiatry 1971; 118: 381-4
39. King RA. Childhood-onset schizophrenia: development and pathogenesis. Child Adolesc Psychiatr Clin North Am 1994; 3 (1): 1-13

40. Gordon CT, Frazier JA, McKenna K, et al. Childhood-onset schizophrenia: an NIMH study in progress. Schizophr Bull 1994; 20 (4): 697-712
41. Werry JS, McClellan JM, Chard L. Childhood and adolescent schizophrenic, bipolar, and schizoaffective disorders: a clinical and outcome study. J Am Acad Child Adolesc Psychiatry 1991; 30: 457-65
42. Remschmidt HE, Schulz E, Martin M, et al. Childhood-onset schizophrenia: history of the concept and recent studies. Schizophr Bull 1994; 20 (4): 727-45
43. Remschmidt H, Martin M, Schulz E, et al. The concept of positive and negative schizophrenia in child and adolescent psychiatry. In: Marneros A, Andreasen NC, Tsuang MT, editors. Negative versus positive schizophrenia. Berlin: Springer-Verlag, 1991: 219-42
44. Asarnow RF, Sherman T. Studies on visual information processing in schizophrenic children. Child Dev 1984; 55: 249-61
45. Asarnow RF, Sherman T, Strandburg R. The search for the psychobiological substrate of childhood onset schizophrenia. J Am Acad Child Psychiatry 1986; 25: 601-14
46. Schneider SG, Asarnow RF. A comparison of cognitive/neuropsychological impairments of nonretarded autistic and schizophrenic children. J Abnorm Child Psychol 1987; 15: 29-45
47. Asarnow RF, Asamen J, Granholm E, et al. Cognitive/neuropsychological studies of children with a schizophrenic disorder. Schizophr Bull 1994; 20 (4): 647-69
48. Alaghband-Rad J, McKenna K, Gordon CT, et al. Childhood-onset schizophrenia: the severity of premorbid course. J Am Acad Child Adolesc Psychiatry 1995; 34 (10): 1273-83
49. Russell AT. The clinical presentation of childhood-onset schizophrenia. Schizophr Bull 1994; 20: 631-46
50. Rosenbaum Asarnow J, Tompson MC, Goldstein MJ. Childhood-onset schizophrenia: a follow-up study. Schizophr Bull 1994; 20 (4): 599-617
51. Caplan R. Childhood schizophrenia assessment and treatment: a developmental approach. Child Adolesc Psychiatr Clin North Am 1994; 3: 15-30
52. Kolvin I, Garside RF, Kidd JSH. Studies in the childhood psychoses: IV. Parental personality and attitude and childhood psychoses. Br J Psychiatry 1971; 118: 403-6
53. Spencer EK, Campbell M. Children with schizophrenia: diagnosis, phenomenology, and pharmacotherapy. Schizophr Bull 1994; 20 (4): 713-25
54. Kydd RR, Werry JS. Schizophrenia in children under 16 years. J Autism Dev Disord 1971; 12: 343-57
55. Rothstein A. Hallucinatory phenomena in childhood. A critique of the literature. J Am Acad Child Psychiatry 1981; 20: 623-35
56. Egdell HG, Kolvin I. Childhood hallucinations. J Child Psychol Psychiatry 1972; 13: 279-87
57. Bender L, Vogel FB. Imaginary companions of children. Am J Orthopsychiatry 1941; 11: 56-65
58. Anthony J. An experimental approach to the psychopathology of childhood: sleep disturbances. Br J Med Psychol 1959; 32: 19-37
59. Despert JL. Delusional and hallucinatory experiences in children. Am J Psychiatry 1948; 104: 528-37
60. Garralda ME. Characteristics of the psychoses of late onset in children and adolescents: a comparative study of hallucinating children. J Adolesc 1985; 8: 195-207
61. Kotsopoulos S, Kaningsberg J, Cote A, et al. Hallucinatory experiences in nonpsychotic children. J Am Acad Child Adolesc Psychiatry 1987; 26: 375-80
62. Propping P. Genetic disorders presenting as 'schizophrenia'. Hum Genet 1983; 65: 1-10
63. Remschmidt H, Martin M. Die Therapie der Schizophrenie im Jugendalter. Dt Ärzteblatt 1992; 89: 387-96
64. Bellack AS, Mueser KT. Psychosocial treatment for schizophrenia. Schizophrenia Bull 1993; 19 (2): 317-36
65. Scott JE, Dixon LB. Psychological interventions for schizophrenia. Schizophrenia Bull 1995; 21 (4): 621-30
66. Harding CM, Zahniser JH. Empirical correction of seven myths about schizophrenia with implications for treatment. Acta Psychiatr Scand 1994; 90 Suppl. 384: 140-6
67. Dixon LB, Lehman AF. Family interventions for schizophrenia. Schizophrenia Bull 1995; 21 (4): 631-43
68. Diamond GS, Serrano AC, Dickey M, et al. Current status of family-based outcome and process research. J Am Acad Child Adolesc Psychiatry 1996; 35 (1): 6-16
69. McClellan J, Werry J. Practice parameters for the assessment and treatment of children and adolescents with schizophrenia. J Am Acad Child Adolesc Psychiatry 1994; 33 (5): 616-35
70. Spencer EK, Kafantaris V, Padron-Gayol M, et al. Haloperidol in schizophrenic children: early findings from a study in progress. Psychopharmacol Bull 1992; 28 (2): 183-6
71. Pool D, Bloom W, Wielke DH, et al. A controlled evaluation of loxitane in seventy-five adolescent schizophrenic patients. Curr Ther Res 1976; 19: 99-104
72. Naruse H, Nagahata M, Nakane Y, et al. A multi-center double-blind trial of pimozide (Orap), haloperidol and placebo in children with behavioral disorders, using a crossover design. Acta Paedopsychiatrica 1982; 48: 173-84
73. Guy W. ECDEU assessment manual for psychopharmacology. Rockville (MD): National Institute of Mental Health, 1976: DHEW Pub No (ADM) 76-338
74. Overall JE, Pfefferbaum B. The brief Psychiatric Rating Scale for Children. Psychopharmacol Bull 1982; 18 (2): 10-6
75. National Institute of Mental Health. Special feature: rating scales and assessment instruments for use in pediatric psycho-pharmacology research. Psychopharmacol Bull 1985; 21 (4): 765-70
76. Coward DM. General pharmacology of clozapine. Br J Psychiatry 1992; 160 Suppl. 17: 5-11
77. Farde L, Nordstrom AL. PET analysis indicates atypical central dopamine receptor occupancy in clozapine-treated patients. Br J Psychiatry 1992; 160 Suppl. 17: 30-3
78. Kuoppamäki M, Syvalahti E, Hietala J. Clozapine and N-desmethylclozapine are potent 5-HT(1C) receptor antagonists. Eur J Pharmacol – Molec Pharm 1993; 245 (2): 179-82

79. Meltzer HY. The importance of serotonin-dopamine interactions in the action of clozapine. Br J Psychiatry 1992; 160 Suppl. 17: 22-9
80. Siefen G, Remschmidt H. Behandlungsergebnisse mit Clozapin bei schizophrenen Jugendlichen. Z Kinder Jugendpsychiat 1986; 14: 245-57
81. Remschmidt H, Schulz E, Martin M. An open trial of clozapine in thirty-six adolescents with schizophrenia. J Child Adolesc Psychopharmacol 1994; 4: 31-41
82. Frazier JA, Gordon CT, McKenna K, et al. An open trial of clozapine in 11 adolescents with childhood-onset schizophrenia. J Am Acad Child Adolesc Psychiatry 1994; 33 (5): 658-63
83. Remschmidt H, Schulz E, Martin M. Die Behandlung schizophener Psychosen in der Adoleszenz mit Clozapin (Leponex). In: Naber D, Müller-Spahn F, editors. Clozapin, Pharmakologie und Klinik eines atypischen Neuroleptikums. Eine kritische Bestandsaufnahme. Stuttgart: Schattauer, 1992: 99-119
84. Mozes T, Toren P, Chernauzan N, et al. Clozapine treatment in very early onset schizophrenia. J Am Acad Child Adolesc Psychiatry 1994; 33 (1): 65-70
85. Birmaher B, Baker R, Kapur S, et al. Clozapine for the treatment of adolescents with schizophrenia. J Am Acad Child Adolesc Psychiatry 1992; 31 (1): 160-4
86. Amminger GP, Resch F, Reimitz J, et al. Nebenwirkungen von Clozapin in der Therapie psychotischer Zustandsbilder bei Jugendlichen. Eine retrospektive klinische Studie. Z Kinder Jugendpsychiat 1992; 20 (1): 5-11
87. Braun-Scharm H, Martinius J. EEG changes and seizures in adolescents with schizophrenia on clozapine [in German]. Z Kinder Jugendpsychiat 1992; 19 (3): 164-9
88. Schulz E, Remschmidt H, Martin M. Clozapin in der Kinder- und Jugendpsychiatrie. In: Naber D, Müller-Spahn F, editors. Clozapin. Pharmakologie und Klinik eines atypischen Neuroleptikums. Berlin: Springer-Verlag, 1994: 23-37
89. Blanz B, Schmidt MH. Clozapine for schizophrenia [letter]. J Am Acad Child Adolesc Psychiatry 1993; 32: 223-4
90. Burke MS, Josephson A, Sebastian CS, et al. Clozapine and cognitive function. J Am Acad Child Adolesc Psychiatry 1995; 34 (2): 127-8
91. Towbin KE, Dykens EM, Pugliese RG. Clozapine for early developmental delays with childhood-onset schizophrenia – protocol and 15-month outcome. J Am Acad Child Adolesc Psychiatry 1994; 33 (5): 651-7
92. Piscitelli SC, Frazier JA, McKenna K, et al. Plasma clozapine and haloperidol concentrations in adolescents with childhood-onset schizophrenia – association with response. J Clin Psychiatry 1994; 55 (9): 94-7
93. Schulz E, Fleischhaker C, Remschmidt H. Determination of clozapine and its major metabolites in serum samples of adolescent schizophrenic patients by high performance liquid chromatography. Data from a prospective clinical trial. Pharmacopsychiatry 1995; 28 (1): 20-5
94. Umbricht D, Kane JM. Risperidone: efficacy and safety. Schizophr Bull 1995; 21 (4): 593-606
95. Fras I, Major LF. Clinical experience with risperidone [letter]. J Am Acad Child Adolesc Psychiatry 1995; 34 (7): 833
96. Cozza SJ, Edison DL. Risperidone in adolescents [letter]. J Am Acad Child Adolesc Psychiatry 1994; 33 (8): 1211
97. Purdon SE, Lit W, Labelle A, et al. Risperidone in the treatment of pervasive developmental disorder. Can J Psychiatry 1994; 39 (7): 400-5
98. Sternlicht HC, Wells SR. Risperidone in childhood schizophrenia [letter]. J Am Acad Child Adolesc Psychiatry 1995; 34 (5): 540
99. McClellan M, Werry JS. Schizophrenia. Pediatric psychopharmacology. Psychiatr Clin North Am 1992; 15 (1): 131-48
100. Campbell M, Spencer EK. Psychopharmacology in child and adolescent psychiatry: a review of the past 5 years. J Am Acad Child Adolesc Psychiatry 1988; 27: 269-79
101. Realmuto GM, Erickson WD, Yellin AM, et al. Clinical comparison of thiothixene and thioridazine in schizophrenic adolescents. Am J Psychiatry 1984; 141: 440-2
102. Richardson MA, Haugland G, Craig TJ. Neuroleptic use, parkinsonian symptoms, tardive dyskinesia, and associated features in child and adolescent psychiatric patients. Am J Psychiatry 1991; 148: 1322-8
103. Rosenberg DR, Holttum J, Gershon S. Textbook of pharmacotherapy for child and adolescent psychiatric disorders. New York: Brunner/Mazel, 1994
104. Campbell M, Grega DM, Green WH, et al. Neuroleptic-induced dyskinesias in children. Clin Neuropharmacol 1983; 6: 207-22
105. Gualtieri CT, Quade D, Hicks RE, et al. Tardive dyskinesia and other clinical consequences of neuroleptic treatment in children and adolescents. Am J Psychiatry 1984; 141: 20-3
106. Gualtieri CT, Schroeder SR, Hicks RE, et al. Tardive dyskinesia in young mentally retarded individuals. Arch Gen Psychiatry 1986; 43: 335-40
107. Silva RR, Magee HJ, Friedhoff AJ. Persistent tardive dyskinesia and other neuroleptic-related dyskinesias in Tourette's disorder. J Child Adolesc Psychopharmacol 1993; 3 (3): 137-44
108. Schooler NR, Kane JM. Research diagnoses for tardive dyskinesia. Arch Gen Psychiatry 1982; 39: 486-7
109. American Psychiatric Association. Task force on late neurological effects of antipsychotic drugs. Tardive dyskinesia: summary of a task force report of the American Psychiatric Association. Am J Psychiatry 1980; 137 (10): 1163-72
110. Green WH. Child and adolescent clinical psychopharmacology. Baltimore: Williams and Wilkins, 1991

Correspondence: Prof. *Helmut Remschmidt*, Department of Child and Adolescent Psychiatry, Philipps University, Hans-Sachs-Str. 6, 35033 Marburg, Germany.

This article is reprinted unchanged from that published originally in *CNS Drugs* 1996; 6: 100-12

Current Drug Therapy Recommendations for the Treatment of Attention Deficit Hyperactivity Disorder

Monica Cyr and *Candace S. Brown*

Department of Pharmacy Practice and Pharmacoeconomics, College of Pharmacy, University of Tennessee, Memphis, Tennessee, USA

1. Attention Deficit Hyperactivity Disorder

1.1 Diagnostic Criteria

Attention deficit hyperactivity disorder (ADHD) is defined by the DSM-IV, as persistent inattentive and/or hyperactive behaviours that are not age-appropriate.[1] These behaviours are pervasive, as demonstrated by their presence in at least two environments (e.g. school and home), and are sufficiently severe so as to interfere with social or academic functioning. To meet DSM-IV criteria, patients must demonstrate symptoms of ADHD before the age of 7 years, and symptoms must have been ongoing for longer than 6 months.

Depending on the symptoms present, ADHD is subclassified as either predominantly inattentive, predominantly hyperactive-impulsive, or both. If at least 6 symptoms of inattentiveness have been present during the previous 6 months, with fewer than 6 symptoms of hyperactivity-impulsivity, then the classification of predominantly inattentive type is made. The converse would qualify for the predominantly hyperactive-impulsive type, whereas the combined type requires at least six symptoms in each category. Symptoms of inattentiveness and hyperactivity-impulsivity as defined in the DSM-IV are listed in table I.

The World Health Organization's International Classification of Disease (ICD-10) recognises these behaviours as hyperkinetic disorder. The ICD construct denotes onset usually before the age of 5, with major areas of impairment being the inability to complete activities requiring concentration or attention, and excessive and indiscriminate motor behaviours. The ICD-10 construct notes that hyperkinetic disorder is commonly associated with delayed motor and language development.[2]

1.2 Aetiology

Numerous aetiological theories based on response to psychostimulants have pointed to lower noradrenaline (norepinephrine) and dopamine turnover, but such a simplistic neuroreceptor theory is unlikely. A more complex theory proposes dopamine dysregulation in the frontal-neostriatal systems which manifests as widely varying states of arousal.[3]

1.3 Incidence

Estimates in the US suggest that ADHD occurs in 3 to 5% of school-age children, and is 4 to 9 times more common in boys than girls.[1] The incidence varies appreciably by country, which may reflect diagnostic constructs, population sampled, and point of view (e.g. physician versus teacher reports).[4-6] Children with first-degree relatives with ADHD are at increased risk for developing ADHD. At least 55% of cases are thought to be inherited, as supported by the 51% concordance rate between monozygotic twins versus a 33% concordance rate between dizygotic twins.[7] Despite the strong evidence supporting a genetic component of ADHD, no specific gene for the disorder has been identified.

Table I. Symptoms of inattention and hyperactivity-impulsivity (from the American Psychiatric Association,[1] with permission)

Inattention

Not attentive to details or makes careless mistakes in schoolwork, work, or other activities

Difficulty sustaining attention in tasks or play activities

Does not seem to listen when spoken to directly

Does not follow through on instructions and fails to finish schoolwork, chores or duties

Has difficulty organising tasks and activities

Avoids, dislikes or is reluctant to engage in tasks that require sustained mental effort

Loses things necessary for tasks or activities

Forgetful in daily activities

Hyperactivity

Often fidgets with hands or feet or squirms in seat

Often leaves seat in classroom or in other situations in which remaining seated is expected

Runs about or climbs excessively in situations in which it is inappropriate

Has difficulty playing or engaging in leisure activities quietly

Often 'on the go' or often acts as if 'driven by a motor'

Talks excessively

Impulsivity

Often blurts out answers before questions have been completed

Has difficulty awaiting turn

Interrupts or intrudes on others

The onset of ADHD usually occurs in toddlerhood (age 2 to 3 years), and its course is not predictable. Symptoms were thought to diminish during late adolescence, but in up to 60% of cases they may persist into adulthood. Factors related to the persistence of symptoms beyond childhood appear to include a family history of ADHD, psychosocial adversity, and comorbid conduct, mood or anxiety disorders.[8,8a]

1.4 Differential Diagnosis and Comorbidity

A thorough mental status examination, input from teachers and family members, and the exclusion of other diagnoses with similar manifestations are crucial to establishing the diagnosis. Symptoms of inattentiveness may result from insufficient sleep, poor nutrition, visual or auditory impairments, or seizures. Anxiety, depression or learning disabilities may sometimes be mistaken for ADHD. Use of prescription medications such as phenobarbital (phenobarbitone) or carbamazepine, or illicit substances including alcohol may also manifest with symptoms of inattentiveness. Impulsive and maladaptive behaviours associated with oppositional defiant disorder also can be mistaken for ADHD. The discriminating factor is that children with oppositional defiant disorder wilfully or angrily resist any behaviour asked of them by an authority figure, whereas ADHD behaviours are not wilfully disobedient. It is estimated that about 40% of children with ADHD also meet criteria for oppositional defiant disorder.[1,9,10]

Conduct disorder is present in at least 21% of children with ADHD, and can manifest in a similar manner to ADHD. Behaviours associated with conduct disorder include aggressiveness or destructiveness, deceitfulness and/or serious infraction of socially accepted norms.[1,9,10]

Overall, children with ADHD have a 25-fold greater risk of institutionalisation for delinquent behaviours, a 5-fold greater risk of drug abuse and a 10-fold greater risk of developing antisocial personality disorder.[10]

2. Psychosocial Interventions

The role of psychosocial interventions in the treatment of ADHD has been the focus of a recently completed 5-year study by the National Institute of Mental Health (NIMH).[11] This randomised, multisite study of 579 participants compared four treatment arms: behavioural interventions, medication management, behavioural interventions combined with medication management, and a community comparison group. Behavioural interventions consisted of teacher and parent training programmes as well as direct interaction between the child and therapist. The medication management arm made use of stimulants as the primary treatment modality with imipramine as a second-line agent for nonresponders. Patients assigned to the community comparison group obtained treatment per their provider without study interference. Treatment was continued for 14 months.

Behavioural interventions provided an effective means of managing symptoms, although the effect sise was not as pronounced as with the medication management group. This may be a consequence of the assessments being completed during medication therapy, but some were obtained months after the behavioural interventions were completed. Three-quarters of the behavioural therapy group were maintained for the duration of the study without pharmacological interventions despite half of the patients receiving medications at the time of randomisation. Behavioural interventions were more acceptable to parents than pharmacological interventions, and appeared to have a greater spectrum of effect on behaviours.

The combination therapy group received 20% less medication at study completion than the medication group, whereas the medication group doses increased by 20% compared with those at initiation. It appears that behavioural approaches continue to be beneficial beyond the intervention stage, whereas medications only provide acute benefits. Behavioural approaches also allow for decreased pharmacological exposure.

3. Pharmacotherapy

3.1 Psychostimulants

Of the pharmacotherapeutic options for treating ADHD, the psychostimulants are the most effective, most commonly used, and most extensively studied. Over 140 studies conducted in primary school–age children (5 to 12 years old) have demonstrated the benefit of stimulants over placebo; a much smaller number of studies have demonstrated their efficacy in other age groups.[12] The stimulants improve hyperactivity, cognition and social interaction. At least 85% of patients respond to one of the three major psychostimulants: methylphenidate, dexamphetamine (dextroamphetamine) or pemoline.[13] A positive response to stimulants should not be used as a means of confirming or establishing the diagnosis of ADHD, as these effects are nonspecific.

The proposed mechanism of action of the stimulants is an increase in catecholamine transmission, particularly dopamine and noradrenaline. Psychostimulants enhance catecholamine transmission via several mechanisms: inhibition of dopamine and noradrenaline reuptake; enhanced presynaptic release of dopamine, noradrenaline and serotonin (5-hydroxytryptamine; 5-HT); and inhibition of monoamine oxidase. The stimulants may have a homeostatic effect which moderates the phasic outbursts of dopaminergic transmission in patients with ADHD.[3,14]

Successful response to the psychostimulants may be affected by comorbid diagnoses. For example, patients with IQ lower than 45 may have a lower response rate, whereas patients with aggression may have a more favourable response.[15,16]

When treating with methylphenidate, attention and concentration are improved at doses of 0.3 mg/kg, and social functioning at doses of 0.6 mg/kg. Peak effects on behaviour occur between 1 and 2 hours postingestion, and diminish within 4 to 6 hours. The dosage should be initiated with 5 to 10mg given after breakfast. Doses can be given two or three times per day, with frequency determined by duration of effect. The second dose is usually given before lunch, and the third before dinner. The dosage can be adjusted weekly according to response, increasing up to the maximum recommended daily dose of 60mg. A sustained-release form requiring only once-daily administration is available, but has lower efficacy than the immediate-release formulation.[17,18]

A new product utilising a once-daily osmotic controlled-release (OROS®) preparation of methylphenidate is expected to be marketed soon. This product is formulated to allow the immediate release of a portion of the dose for rapid onset of effect, as well as provide continuous, controlled drug delivery for a 12-hour duration of effect with a tapering dose at the end of the day.[18a] A daily transdermal formulation of methylphenidate is poised to enter phase III trials later this year. It is expected that the transdermal route may decrease typical adverse effects of oral administration.[18b] These new pharmaceutical dosage forms are likely to provide effective and convenient alternatives to currently available methylphenidate formulations.

Subtleties in mechanisms of action among the stimulants allow for response to one stimulant despite nonresponse to another. Dexamphetamine is as effective as methylphenidate and is often used in the event of an inadequate response to the latter. The longer duration of effect of dexamphetamine minimises breakthrough symptoms while allowing for less frequent administration. These benefits are often outweighed by its greater incidence of anorexia and growth suppression, and higher abuse potential. Dexamphetamine should be initiated with a 5mg daily dosage and titrated upwards in 5mg increments weekly. The maximum recommended daily dose is 40mg.

A combination of four amphetamine salts previously marketed for weight reduction has recently been targeted for use in the ADHD population. This product provides a 3:1 ratio of dextro- and levo-isomers of amphetamine, and is marketed under the name Adderall®. Its efficacy has been demonstrated clinically, and it appears to have a comparable adverse effect profile to methylphenidate. It is more potent than methylphenidate, and its peak and duration of effect appear to be dose related. Although twice-daily administration may be necessary in some cases, symptoms in most patients appear to be well controlled with morning administration only. Adderall® also appears to be effective in patients with symptoms previously nonresponsive to methylphenidate.[21a-d]

Because of the increased potential for hepatotoxicity, pemoline is usually reserved for patients who do not respond to either stimulants. Pemoline is administered once daily, and traditional dosage regimens have advised gradual upward titration from 18.75mg to achieve effect. On the premise that pemoline had a delayed onset of action, increments of 18.75mg were advised every 3 to 4 weeks. Pelham et al.[19] have studied the time- and dose-response curves of pemoline, and have determined that onset of effect occurs within 2 hours after ingestion and lasts for 7 hours. Thus, it has been suggested that pemoline be initiated at 37.5 to 56.25mg daily, with dose increments to be made every 2 to 3 days. When administered at a pemoline 6mg : methylphenidate 1mg ratio, pemoline has the same efficacy as methylphenidate.[17,19]

Of patients receiving pemoline, 1 to 2% develop hepatotoxicity. Elevations in liver function tests (LFTSs) may occur as soon as 6 months after initiation of therapy and as late as 5 years.[20,20a] One case of hepatotoxicity occurred 5 weeks after reinitiating pemoline.[20] Elevations in LFTs usually return to baseline within 2 to 9 months of discontinuing pemoline, but two fatalities resulting from fulminant failure have been reported.[20b,20c] The relative risk is calculated to be 45 times greater than that associated with the other stimulants.[21] It is often recommended that LFTs be monitored every 6 months. As onset of hepatitis may occur during any point in therapy, it is equally important to educate the patient and family about the manifestations of liver failure such as fatigue, jaundice, nausea or vomiting.

All stimulants share the same adverse effect profile, with the most common adverse events being decreased appetite (41%), headache (10%), irritability (26%), insomnia (28%) and gastrointestinal irritability (23%). These tend to be more pronounced when initiating therapy or increasing the dose, and tend to decrease with time. Anorexia and gastrointestinal irritability may be minimised by administration with or after meals. Headaches may be relieved by decreasing the dose, but may necessitate a change in therapy. Irritability or dysphoria may respond to a dose decrease, but in some cases may require a switch to another stimulant or to an antidepressant. Although insomnia may occur as an adverse effect of stimulant use, it may be a manifestation of ADHD symptoms or a rebound effect due to the short duration of action of the stimulant (in particular methylphenidate). Other possible causes of insomnia should be identified and addressed. Administering the last dose of stimulant earlier in the day will alleviate insomnia if it is an actual adverse effect, whereas administering a small dose of stimulant close to bedtime will improve insomnia if the difficulty stems from ADHD symptoms or withdrawal.[22]

An adverse effect of some concern is growth suppression. Treatment of ADHD with stimulants has been associated with small but statistically significant decreases in bodyweight and height which do not appear to be clinically significant. Furthermore, children receiving stimulants have not demonstrated bodyweight or height reduction persisting into adulthood.[23] Attempts to minimise growth suppression by using drug holidays during the summer months may allow for a 'catch-up' period of growth. Drug holidays should not be considered an absolute requirement, as they may not be acceptable for children who have significant functional impairment.[24] Dexamphetamine may be the stimulant most likely to cause growth retardation.[25]

Another adverse effect of concern and controversy while treating with stimulants is the potential for developing tics. It is generally accepted that tic disorders can be a contraindication to the use of stimulants, although the clinical basis for this recommendation is equivocal.

Stimulants have been reported to unmask or increase the severity or number of tics in some patients,[26] and to ameliorate them in others.[27,28] Evidence which suggests a genetic relationship between ADHD and Tourette's syndrome[29] further complicates the issue. At the current time, the more prudent approach appears to be to avoid the use of psychostimulants if the tricyclic antidepressants (TCAs) or clonidine can be used successfully in patients with concomitant tic disorders. If alternative therapies are not successful, use of the stimulants with careful monitoring for tic exacerbation appears to be an appropriate strategy.

Possible tolerance, dependence and abuse of stimulants is often of concern to parents, pharmacists and practitioners. The literature bears little support for the development of tolerance or dependence. If tolerance appears to be occurring, it is important to rule out possible noncompliance before changing to another formulation or agent. Abuse by the patient, family or patient's peers are legitimate concerns that must be taken into consideration, but should not prevent patients from obtaining adequate therapy. Although under-recognition and under-reporting of abuse is a fair assumption, only four cases have been published.[29a-c] Nevertheless, ADHD is associated with a greater risk of significant drug abuse following experimentation with drugs when compared with non-ADHD peers.[29d]

3.2 Tricyclic Antidepressants

Over 25 studies, mostly of imipramine and desipramine, have been conducted in primary school–age children to establish the efficacy of TCAs in treating ADHD.[12] These agents do not appear to provide as much benefit in treating the cognitive symptoms of ADHD as the stimulants, but are considered second-line agents for patients who do not respond adequately to the latter.[24,30] They may be most beneficial for patients with ADHD and a concomitant anxiety or tic disorder.[31] However, monotherapy with TCAs in treating ADHD in depressed patients may not provide adequate antidepressant coverage. Of the 11 double-blind, controlled trials assessing the antidepressant effects of the TCAs in children and adolescents, 10 have shown no antidepressant effect.[32]

TCAs must be given twice daily in children due to their more rapid metabolism and resultant shorter half-life. The first dose is usually given in the morning and the second dose at bedtime. Administration of drugs such as imipramine and desipramine should be initiated with 10mg twice daily, and titrated upwards every 5 days to 3 mg/kg. Daily doses of up to 5 mg/kg may be administered. There is no established plasma concentration-response relationship, but routine plasma concentrations should be monitored to minimise the toxic potential.[12,22]

The benefits of TCAs over the stimulants include lack of need for drug administration during school hours, fewer disruptions to sleep, appetite and growth patterns, no rebound effects, low abuse potential, and no negative effects on tic disorders. However, unlike the stimulants, tolerance to the therapeutic effects may develop over time.

The use of TCAs requires that careful attention be paid to the potential for overdose, lowering of seizure threshold and adverse cardiac effects. A baseline

Table II. Electocardiographic parameters of concern in children receiving tricyclic antidepressants[37]

PR interval > 200 msec
QRS interval > 30% above baseline
QRS interval > 120 msec
QT$_c$ interval > 480 msec
Systolic blood pressre > 120mm Hg
Diastolic blood pressure > 80mm Hg
Heart rate > 130 beats/min at rest

EEG should be obtained in patients with a history of seizures or head trauma. Seven cases of sudden death have been reported in children receiving desipramine.[33-36] A baseline electrocardiogram (ECG) should be obtained, and should be repeated after steady-state has been achieved. Guidelines for the discontinuation of tricyclics based on ECG monitoring are presented in table II.[37]

3.3 Monoamine Oxidase Inhibitors

On the basis of the monoamine oxidase inhibition effects of the stimulants, the monoamine oxidase inhibitor (MAOI) antidepressants tranylcypromine, clorgiline (clorgyline), moclobemide and selegiline (deprenyl) have been studied in this patient population.[38-42,42a] Results have shown moderate to robust response, but only one study was controlled. These agents are not popular options due to the need for maintaining a low-tyramine diet when treating with the nonreversible MAOIs, and their use is not supported by the literature.

3.4 Amfebutamone (Bupropion)

Six double-blind studies[43-48] have been conducted to assess efficacy in children with ADHD. All but one[47] yielded positive results. Amfebutamone seems to be a promising antidepressant alternative for the treatment of ADHD. It is neither associated with cardiac conduction abnormalities,[49] nor does it have potential for abuse.[50] Nonetheless, amfebutamone has been reported to exacerbate tics,[51,52] and may increase the risk of seizures in patients with seizure disorders.[22] The drug should be initiated with 50mg twice daily and increased to 125mg twice daily over two weeks. Common adverse effects include dry mouth, insomnia, headaches and tremors.

3.5 Selective Serotonin Reuptake Inhibitors

No systematic studies are available to assess the efficacy of selective serotonin reuptake inhibitors (SSRIs) in patients with ADHD. Two open-label studies of fluoxetine have demonstrated moderate success in children,[53,54] and a case-study of sertraline in a 24-year-old woman with ADHD suggests efficacy without exacerbation of her tic disorder.[55] At this time, there is not sufficient support for the use of the SSRIs in the treatment of ADHD.

3.6 Antipsychotics

Antipsychotics have been shown to decrease hyperactivity in children with ADHD, but worsen attention and concentration. Effects on learning and cognitive functioning are often deterrents to the use of antipsychotics in this population. Currently available studies are dated and include confounding diagnoses. Given the potential for developing extrapyramidal symptoms, and the lack of evidence supporting improved cognition, the antipsychotics are not recommended for the treatment of ADHD.[12]

3.7 Clonidine

Clonidine is an α_2 noradrenergic agonist which is most commonly used as an adjunctive agent for patients with inadequate response to stimulants alone. Three controlled studies have been conducted in children with ADHD.[56-58] behavioural improvements were reported in all studies, with fewer effects on cognition. The maximum dosage is 0.3 µg/kg/day divided into

3 or 4 doses. To minimise adverse effects, administration should be initiated with 0.05mg at bedtime. Slow titration and onset of effect delays maximal effects for several months. The patch formulation may be used to enhance compliance, but it may not adhere well in humid conditions.[10]

Clonidine is associated with sedation and anticholinergic adverse effects which may persist for 3 to 4 weeks. The hypotensive, orthostatic and delayed cardiac conduction effects of clonidine require routine monitoring of these parameters, especially when the dose is increased.

Four cases of sudden death have been reported in children receiving clonidine with either dexamphetamine or methylphenidate. A potential causal relationship is clouded by existing cardiac abnormalities, concurrent medications and anesthesia. Adverse cardiac effects not resulting in death have been reported with the use of clonidine and methylphenidate.[59]

4. Behavioural Assessments

Assessment of medication response based on a glimpse of the child's behaviour in the office may not be representative of the true picture. The new environment and individual attention paid to the child may result in more controlled behaviour. In order to objectify the child's behaviour across settings, it is necessary to rely on both family and teacher rating scales. Observations in the school setting offer a more practical assessment of the child's symptoms as the teacher is able to observe the child across a number of situations and can compare his/her behaviour with non-ADHD children.

Several rating scales have been developed to objectify ADHD behaviours.[10,60] The most commonly used and best validated ones will be reviewed here. The Conners' Teacher Rating Scale (CTRS) is a 28-item assessment with a 48-item parental version, the Conners Parent Questionnaire (CPQ).[61] Both make measurements on a 4-point scale, and each requires about 10 minutes to complete. Achenbach's Child Behavior Checklist[62] is a commonly used parental rating scale which not only detects changes in hyperactive behaviour, but also recognises depressive, aggressive and somatic complaints which can occur concomitantly. The Child Attention Problems (CAP) instrument,[63] derived from the Teacher Report Form (TRF) of the Child Behavior Checklist,[64] is a 12-item, teacher-rated scale designed to reflect changes in behaviour in response to medication. The CAP is usually administered weekly.

In using these rating scales, it is important to remember that the teacher-rated scales tend to provide a more accurate overview of the child's behaviour than the parent-rated scales. A large disparity between the two scales, with the parent-rated scale suggesting worse behaviour, may reflect the child's behavioural reactions to family conflict. A 'halo effect', which may reflect the rater's perception of overall behaviours as opposed to specific ADHD symptoms, may result in the rater rating the child more positively or more negatively on all items, on the basis of behaviours which provide a less discriminating assessment of areas of progress. This may be especially important when comorbidity includes oppositional defiant disorder or conduct disorder.

5. Conclusions and Treatment Recommendations

ADHD affects about 5% of school-age children, impairing their social and academic functioning. Potential long term morbidity includes persistence of symptoms into adulthood, increased risk of antisocial behaviours and increased risk of substance abuse.

Therapy relies on pharmacological methods, as the benefit of psychosocial interventions is not yet clear. The psychostimulants are the agents of choice in most cases. The choice of stimulant is based on potential for adverse effects, rather than efficacy. Pemoline carries the greatest risk of causing liver failure, and is usually relegated to third position. The greater risk of abuse and growth suppression may force dexamphetamine into second place if the child or family members have problems with substance abuse. Whichever stimulant is used, the goal is to enhance academic and social functioning while minimising adverse effects. On the basis of clinical experience, clonidine is often used as an adjunctive agent to the stimulants. Clonidine is not as effective in improving cognitive symptoms of ADHD when used as mono-therapy. Four deaths have been reported with the use of clonidine and methylphenidate, and the combination should be used with caution until the causal relationship can be clarified.

The TCAs are often used as second-line agents when there is an inadequate response or relative contraindication to using stimulants (e.g. tic exacerbation, patient or parental stimulant abuse). To minimise cardiotoxicity, ECGs should be obtained before the start of therapy, during the titration phase, once the target dose is achieved and periodically thereafter. Use of imipramine over desipramine may also be a prudent means of minimising the risk of sudden death. Tolerance to the therapeutic effects of the tricyclics may occur.

Amfebutamone appears to be a viable alternative to the abovementioned modalities, but should be used with caution in patients with tic disorders, seizures or eating disorders. Other antidepressants such as the MAOIs and the SSRIs have not been studied extensively in this population and cannot be recommended at this time.

Antipsychotic agents decrease hyperactivity associated with ADHD, but may negatively effect cognition. Due to their less than optimal therapeutic effects and the potential for extra-pyramidal symptoms, antipsychotics should be avoided in this patient population.

To best evaluate the benefits of therapeutic interventions, objective input should be obtained using parent and teacher rating scales.

References

1. American Psychiatric Association. Attention-deficit and disruptive behavior disorders. In: American Psychiatric Association. Diagnostic and statistical manual of mental disorders. 4th ed. Washington, DC: American Psychiatric Association, 1994: 78-85
2. World Health Organization. Mental and behavioural disorders. In: International statistical classification of disease and related health problems. Vol. 1. 10th rev. Geneva: World Health Organization, 1992: 378-9
3. Evans RW, Gaultieri CT, Hicks RE. A neuropathic substrate for stimulant drug effects in hyperactive children. Clin Neuropharmacol 1986; 9: 264-81
4. Prendergast M, Taylor E, Rapoport JL, et al. The diagnosis of childhood hyperactivity: a U.S.-U.K. cross-national study of DSM-III and ICD-9. J Child Psychol Psychiatry 1988; 29: 289-300
5. Szatmari P, Offord DR, Boyle MH. Ontario child health study: prevalence of attention deficit disorder with hyperactivity. J Child Psychol Psychiatry 1989; 30: 219-30
6. Baumgaertel A, Wolraich ML, Dietrich M. Comparison of diagnostic criteria for attention deficit disorders in a German elementary school sample. J Am Acad Child Adolesc Psychiatry 1995; 34: 629-38
7. Goodman R, Stevenson J. A twin study of hyperactivity: II. The aetiologic role of genes, family relationships, and perinatal adversity. J Child Psychol Psychiatry 1989; 30: 691-709
8. Cantwell DP. Hyperactive children have grown up: what have we learned about what happens to them? Arch Gen Psychiatry 1985; 42: 1026-8
8a. Biederman J, Faraone S, Milberger S, et al. Predictors of persistence and remission of ADHD into adolescence. Results from a four-year propective follow-up study. J Am Acad Child Adolesc Psychiaty 1996; 35: 343-51
9. Searight HR, Nahlik JE, Campbell DC. Attention-deficit/hyperactivity disorder: assessment, diagnosis, and management. J Fam Pract 1995; 40: 270-9
10. American Academy of Child and Adolescent Psychiatry. Practice parameters for the assessment and treatment of children, adolescents, and adults with attention-deficit/hyperactivity disorder. J Am Acad Child Adolesc Psychiatry 1997; 36 (10 Suppl.): 85-121S
11. Pelham WE. The NIMH multimodal treatment study for attention-deficit hyperactivity disorder: just say yes to drugs alone? Can J Psychiatr 1999; 44: 981-90

12. Spencer T, Biederman J, Wilens T, et al. Pharmacotherapy of attention-deficit hyperactivity disorder across the life cycle. J Am Acad Child Adolesc Psychiatry 1996; 35: 409-32

13. Elia J, Borcherding BG, Rapoport JL, et al. Methylphenidate and dextroamphetamine treatments of hyperactivity: are there true nonresponders? Psychiatry Res 1991; 36: 141-55

14. Jacobvitz D, Sroufe LA, Stewart M, et al. Treatment of attentional and hyperactivity problems in children with sympathomimetic drugs: a comprehensive review. J Am Acad Child Adolesc Psychiatry 1990; 29: 677-88

15. Livingston RL, Dykman RA, Ackerman PT. Psychiatric comorbidity and response to two doses of methylphenidate in children with attention deficit disorder. J Child Adolesc Psychopharmacol 1992; 2: 115-22

16. Aman MF, Marks RE, Turbott SH, et al. Clinical effects of methylphenidate and thioridazine in intellectually subaverage children. J Am Acad Child Adolesc Psychiatry 1992; 30: 246-56

17. Pelham WE, Greenslade KE, Vodde-Hamilton M, et al. Relative efficacy of long-acting stimulants on children with ADHD: a comparison of standard methylphenidate, sustained-release methylphenidate, sustained-release dextroamphetamine, and pemoline. Pediatrics 1990; 86: 226-37

18. Fitzpatrick PA, Klorman R, Brumaghim JT, et al. Effects of sustained-release and standard preparations of methylphenidate on attention deficit disorder. J Am Acad Child Adolesc Psychiatry 1992; 31: 226-34

18a. Modi NB, Lindemulder B, Gupta S. Single- and multiple-dose pharmacokinetics of an oral once-a-day osmotic controlled-release OROS® (methylphenidate Hcl) formulation. J Clin Pharmacol 2000; 40: 379-88

18b. FDC Reports. The NDA Pipeline. www.ndapipeline.com. 7-21-00

19. Pelham WE, Swanson JM, Furman MB, et al. Pemoline effects on children with ADHD: a time-response by dose-response analysis on classroom measures. J Am Acad Child Adolesc Psychiatry 1995; 34: 1504-13

20. Rosh JR, Dellert SF, Narkewicz M, et al. Four cases of severe hepatotoxicity associated with pemoline: possible auto-immune pathogenesis. Pediatrics 1998; 101: 921-3

20a. Pratt DS, Dubois RS. Hepatotoxicity due to pemoline (Cylert): a report of two cases. J Pediatr Gastroenterol Nutr 1990; 10: 239-41

20b. Berkovitch M, Pope E, Phillips J, et al. Pemoline-associated fulminant liver failure: testing the evidence for causation. Clin Pharmacol Ther 1995; 57: 696-8

20c. Avery JK. Failure to monitor. Tenn Med 1997: 90 (8): 311-12

21a. Swanson JM, Wigal S, Greenhill LL, et al. Analog classroom assessment of Adderall® in children with ADHD. J Am Acad Child Adolesc Psychiatry 1998; 37: 519-26

21b. Manos MJ, Short EJ, Findling RL. Differential effectiveness of methylphenidate and Adderall® in school-age youths with attention-deficit/hyperactivity disorder. J Am Acad Child Adolesc Psychiatry 1999; 38: 813-19

21c. Pliszka SR, Browne RG, Olvera RL, et al. A double-blind, placebo-controlled study of Adderall and methylphenidate in the treatment of attention-deficit/hyperactivity disorder. J Am Acad Child Adolesc Psychiatry 2000; 39: 619-26

21d. Pelham WE, Aronoff HR, Midlam JK, et al. A comparison of Ritalin and Adderall: efficacy and time-course in children with attention-deficit/hyperactiviy disorder. Pediatrics 1999; 103: e43

21. Berkovitch M, Pope E, Phillips J, et al. Pemoline-associated fulminant liver failure: testing the evidence for causation. Clin Pharmacol Ther 1995; 57: 696-8

22. Bezchlibnyk-Butler KZ, Jeffries JJ, editors. Clinical handbook of psychotropic drugs. Toronto: Hogrefe & Huber, 1996

23. Klein RG, Mannuzza S. Hyperactive boys almost grown up: methylphenidate effects on ultimate height. 1998; 45: 1127-30

24. Spencer TJ, Biederman J, Harding M, et al. Growth deficits in ADHD children revisited: evidence for disorder-associated growth delays? J Am Acad Child Adolesc Psychiatry 1996; 35: 1460-9

25. Greenhill LL. Stimulant-related growth inhibition in children: a review. In: Gittleman M, editor. Strategic interventions for hyperactive children. New York: ME Sharp, 1981: 39-63

26. Lowe TL, Cohen DJ, Detlor J, et al. Stimulant medications precipitate Tourette's syndrome. JAMA 1982; 247: 1729-31

27. Erenberg G, Cruse RP, Rothner AD. Gilles de la Tourette's syndrome: effects of stimulant drugs. Neurology 195; 35: 1346-8

28. Sverd J, Gadow KD, Paolicelli LM. Methylphenidate treatment of attention-deficit hyperactivity disorder in boys with Tourette's syndrome. J Am Acad Child Adolesc Psychiatr 1989; 28: 574-9

29. Knell ER, Comings DE. Tourette's syndrome and attention-deficit hyperactivity disorder: evidence for a genetic relationship. J Clin Psychiatry 1993; 54: 331-7

29a. Goyer PF, Davis GC, Rapaport JL. Abuse of prescribed stimulant medication by a 13-year-old hyperactive boy. J Am Acad Child Adolesc Psychiatry 1979; 18: 170-5

29b. Jaffe SL. Intranasal abuse of prescirbed methylphenidate by an alcohol and drug abusing adolescent with ADHD. J Am Acad Child Adolesc Psychiatry 1991; 30: 773-5

29c. Fulton A, Yates WR. Family abuse of methylphenidate. Am Fam Physician 1988; 38: 143-5

29d. Mannuzza S, Klein RG, Bonagura N, et al. Hyperactive boys almost grown up: II. Status of subjects without mental disorder. Arch Gen Psychiatry 1988; 45: 77-83

30. Pliszka SR. Tricyclic antidepressants in the treatment of children with attention deficit disorder. J Amer Acad Child Adolesc Psychiatry 1987; 26: 127-32

31. Kutcher SP, Reiter S, Gardner DM, et al. The pharmacotherapy of anxiety disorders in children and adolescents. Psychiatr Clin North Am 1992; 15: 41-57

32. Birmaher B, Ryan ND, Williamson DE, et al. Childhood and adolescent depression: a review of the past 10 years. Part II. J Amer Acad Child Adolesc Psychiatry 1996; 35: 1575-83

33. Riddle MA, Nelson JC, Kleinman CS, et al. Sudden death in children receiving Norpramin®: a review of three reported cases and commentary. J Am Acad Child Adolesc Psychiatry 1991; 30: 104-8

34. Riddle MA, Geller B, Ryan N. Another sudden death in a child treated with desipramine. J Am Acad Child Adolesc Psychiatry 1993; 32: 792-7
35. Popper CW, Zimnitzky B. Sudden death putatively related to desipramine treatment in youth: a fifth case and a review of speculative mechanisms. J Child Adolesc Psychopharmacol 1995; 5: 283-300
36. Varley CK, McClellan J. Case study: two additional sudden deaths with tricyclic antidepressants. J Am Acad Child Adolesc Psychiatry 1997; 36: 390-4
37. Wilens TE, Biederman J, Baldessarini RJ, et al. Cardiovascular effects of therapeutic doses of tricyclic antidepressants in children and adolescents. J Am Acad Child Adolesc Psychiatry 1996; 35: 1491-501
38. Priest RG, Gimbrett R, Roberts M, et al. Reversible and selective inhibitors of monoamine oxidase A in mental and other disorders. Acta Psychiatrica Scandinavica 1995; 386: 40-3
39. Trott GE, Friese HJ, Menzel M, et al. Use of moclobemide in children with attention deficit hyperactivity disorder. Jugendpsychiat 1991; 19: 248-53
40. Zametkin A, Rapoport JL, Murphy DL, et al. Treatment of hyperactive children with monoamine oxidase inhibitors: I. Clinical efficacy. Arch Gen Psychiatry 1985; 42; 962-6
41. Wender PH, Wood DR, Reimherr F, et al. An open trial of pargyline in the treatment of attention deficit disorder, residual type. Psychiatry Res 1983; 9: 329-36
42. Wood D, Reimherr F, Wender P. The use of l-deprenyl in the treatment of attention deficit disorder, residual type. Presented at the American College of Neuropsychopharmacology, 1982, San Juan, Puerto Rico
42a. Jankovic J. Deprenyl in attention deficit associated with Tourette's syndrome. Arch Neurol 1993; 50: 286-8
43. Conners CK, Casat CD, Gualtieri CT, et al. Bupropion hydrochloride in attention deficit disorder with hyperactivity. J Am Acad Child Adolesc Psychiatry 1996; 35: 1314-21
44. Clay TH, Gualtieri CT, Evans RW, et al. Clinical and neuropsychological effects of the novel antidepressant bupropion. Psychopharmacol Bull 1988; 24; 143-8
45. Casat CD, Pleasants DZ, Schroeder DH, et al. Bupropion in children with attention deficit disorder. Psychopharmacol Bull 1989; 25: 198-201
46. Casat CD, Pleasants DZ, Van Wyck Fleet J. A double-blind trial of bupropion in children with attention deficit disorder. Psychopharmacol Bull 1987; 23: 120-2
47. Wolfe KD, Weller EB, Weller RA, et al. Treating children with attention-deficit disorder: a double-blind trial. Presented at the 40th Annual Meeting of the American Academy of Child and Adolescent Psychiatry; 1993; San Antonio (TX)
48. Barrickman LL, Perry PJ, Allen AJ, et al. Bupropion versus methylphenidate in the treatment of attention-deficit hyperactivity disorder. J Am Acad Child Adolesc Psychiatry 1995; 34: 649-57
49. Roose SP, Glassman AH, Giardina EGV, et al. Cardiovascular effects of imipramine and bupropion in depressed patients with congestive heart failure. Am J Psychiatry 1991; 148: 512-6
50. Griffith JD, Griffith C, Carranza J, et al. Bupropion: clinical assay for amphetamine-like abuse potential. J Clin Psychiatry 1983; 44: 206-8
51. Jacobsen LK, Chappell P, Woolston JL. Bupropion and compulsive behavior. J Am Acad Child Adolesc Psychiatry 1994; 33: 143-4
52. Spencer T, Biederman J, Steingard R, et al. Bupropion exacerbates tics in children with attention-deficit hyperactivity disorder and Tourette's syndrome. J Am Acad Child Adolesc Psychiatry 1993; 32: 211-4
53. Barrickman L, Nayes R, Kuperman S, et al. Treatment of ADHD with fluoxetine: a preliminary trial. J Am Acad Child Adolesc Psychiatry 1991; 305: 762-7
54. Campbell NB, Tamburrino MB, Evans CL, et al. Fluoxetine for ADHD in a young child. J Am Acad Child Adolesc Psychiatry 1995; 34: 1259-60
55. Frankenburg FOR, Kando JC. Sertraline treatment of attention deficit hyperactivity disorder and Tourette's syndrome. J Clin Psychopharmacol 1994; 14: 359-60
56. Gunning B. A controlled trial of clonidine in hyperkinetic children [thesis]. Department of Child and Adolescent Psychiatry, Academic Hospital Rotterdam, Sophia Children's Hospital Rotterdam, 1992
57. Hunt RD, Minderaa RB, Cohen DJ. Clonidine benefits children with attention deficit disorder and hyperactivity: report of a double-blind placebo-crossover therapeutic trial. J Am Acad Child Psychiatry 1985; 24: 617-29
58. Hunt Rd, Minderaa RB, Cohen DJ. Therapeutic effect of clonidine in attention deficit disorder with hyperactivity: a comparison with placebo and methylphenidate. Psychopharmacol Bull 1986; 22: 229-36
59. Cantwell DP, Swanson J, Connor DF. Case study: adverse response to clonidine. J Am Acad Child Psychiatry 1997; 36: 539-44
60. Edlebrock CS, Rancurello MD. Childhood hyperactivity: an overview of rating scales and their applications. Clin Psychol Rev 1985; 5: 429-45
61. Conners CK. A teacher rating scale for use in drug studies with children. Am J Psychiatry 1969; 126; 884-8
62. Achenbach TM. Integrative guide for the 1991 CBCL/4-18, YSR, and TRF profiles. Burlington: University of Vermont Department of Psychiatry, 1991
63. Barkley RA. Attention deficit hyperactivity disorder: a handbook for diagnosis and treatment. New York: Guilford, 1990
64. Achenbach TM. Manual for the Teacher's Report Form and 1991 Profile. Burlington: University of Vermont Department of Psychiatry, 1991

Correspondence: Dr *Monica Cyr*, Department of Pharmacy Practice and Pharmacoeconomics, College of Pharmacy, University of Tennessee, 847 Monroe Avenue, Memphis, TN 38163, USA.

Therapeutics of Aggression in Children

Daniel S. Pine and *Elizabeth Cohen*

Division of Child Psychiatry, New York State Psychiatric Institute, Columbia University College of Physicians and Surgeons, New York, New York, USA

While the term 'aggression' has been used to describe a variety of behaviours in a diverse array of species, this review focuses on the treatment of aggression as a manifestation of mental illness in children. The term 'aggression' is defined as behaviour intended to harm another individual. While the current review will emphasise the use of drug therapy in children (individuals below the age of 18 years) with mental illness, this discussion will be placed within the broader context of current knowledge on the clinical characteristics and multimodal treatment of paediatric aggression.

Research reports forming the basis for the current literature review were generated from a computer-based literature search using both *Medline* and *PsychInfo* to locate all potentially relevant articles published in the past 20 years. The terms for these searches were as follows: aggression; disruptive behaviour; conduct disorder (CD); attention deficit hyperactivity disorder (ADHD); and oppositional defiant disorder (ODD). Each of these terms was conjoined with either 'child' or 'adolescent' as key words. Abstracts for all articles and the full text of all potentially relevant articles were reviewed. This information was supplemented with a review of other articles located either from the reference lists of the reviewed articles or from the reference lists from reviews or chapters in major textbooks on the topic.

1. Phenomenology

The most common psychiatric problems in children are separated into two broad categories: internalising syndromes, which include anxiety and mood disorders; and externalising syndromes, which include the three disruptive behaviour disorders from the DSM-IV: ADHD, ODD and CD.[1,2] Aggression can arise in many clinical scenarios, including as part of internalising, externalising, or other syndromes. For example, children with pervasive developmental disorders can exhibit problems with aggressive behaviour. Similarly, there has been a particularly increasing interest in the association between aggression and possible variants of bipolar disorder, an internalising syndrome.[3] Since many therapeutic studies target aggression that arises as part of a disruptive behaviour disorder,[1,4] the current review focuses on aggression accompanying each of these syndromes. Nevertheless, it is crucial to consider the full range of diagnoses examined in any study on the treatment of paediatric aggression, as children with different diagnoses may exhibit unique responses to various interventions. As reviewed below, the majority of pharmacological treatment studies on paediatric aggression target children with disruptive behaviour disorders.

DSM-IV recognises the disruptive disorders as three unique conditions based on differences in phenomenology, risk factors and course.[1,5,6] ADHD is characterised by a triad of inattentive, hyperactive and impulsive behaviour; ODD is characterised by a pattern of recurrent hostility, defiance and refusal to comply; CD is characterised by recurrent aggression and rule violations. Despite the unique features of these three syndromes, treatment often targets aggression and tends to be similar for each condition.[1,7-10] In fact, some investigators question the degree of distinction among the three syndromes.[1,4,6-8] Biological and treatment data provide some support for this view.[6,7]

As reviewed by Vitiello and Stoff,[11] childhood aggression has been categorised into various forms using an array of criteria. For example, aggression can be categorised based on phenomenology into so-called emotive as opposed to predatory aggression. Alternatively, early and late onset variants of aggressive behaviour problems have been distinguished based on the unique course and neuropsychological profile across these two variants.[4] Others have focused on the overt or covert nature of aggression.

Despite the various methods for categorising paediatric aggression, treatment studies rely on relatively consistent measurement strategies. Typically, standardised questionnaires are administered to parents and teachers inquiring about details on the number and severity of aggressive episodes. Two commonly used measures include the rating scales developed by Conners[12] and Achenbach et al.[1] Other studies have relied on direct observations and ratings of aggressive acts, as described in the Overt Aggression Scale of Yudofsky et al.[13] Despite the current interest in variants of aggressive behaviour, most treatment studies consider effects on global ratings of aggression. In future studies, Vitiello and Stoff[11] suggest that pharmacological interventions might be targeted at children with more impulsive or emotive forms of aggression. It has been noted in basic science studies that pharmacological interventions might specifically target emotive aggression. Psychotherapy, on the other hand, might be especially useful in children with planned aggression.

From the developmental perspective, aggression represents one of the most persistent childhood psychiatric problems. Prospective studies find as large a correlation across development for aggressive behaviour as for intelligence.[14,15] Aggression that arises before puberty is thought to be particularly stable and severe.[4] The form of this longitudinal association suggests the importance of research on distinguishing transient from persistent aggression in children – most adults with chronic aggression have a history of aggression since childhood, though many aggressive children become nonaggressive as they age.[8,9,16]

Studies on the individual disruptive behaviour disorders suggest a developmental progression, such that individuals with lifelong histories of aggression initially show signs of irritability, hostility and temper outbursts as young children.[10,17] Symptoms consistent with ADHD are most observable during school age, which progress to symptoms of ODD. These symptoms, in turn, can develop into CD. Finally, while prospective studies clearly delineate a high degree of stability in aggression, this consistent level of aggression across development is manifested in ratings of behaviour that summarise relatively long periods of time, in the order of weeks to a few months. On a day-to-day basis, aggressive behaviour tends to be episodic, even among highly aggressive children.

2. The Aetiology of Aggression

Aggression arising as part of a disruptive behaviour disorder generally develops in one of two clinical scenarios. As children enter adolescence there are marked increases in aggressive and oppositional behaviour, such that some children first develop problems with aggression as adolescents.[4] Other children exhibit aggression during childhood, often as part of ADHD, which then develops into symptoms of CD before adolescence. This second pattern has been labelled 'lifelong persistent' aggression. This review focuses on theories of lifelong persistent aggression, as this pattern is most clinically impairing and persistent, is seen most frequently by clinicians and is most closely tied to biological abnormalities.[4]

Earlier research on the ogy of chronic aggression focused on single domains of risk.[18] Hence, one body of research explored environmental factors, while another focused on biology. As evidence accumulated, theories focusing on only environmental or biological factors received less support than theories emphasising the interplay between biological and environmental factors. We briefly summarise earlier research on single domains of risk before describing more recent studies examining the interplay between domains.

Environmental risk factors can be conceived at many levels, from the societal level to the level of parent-child interactions. At the societal level, neighbourhood factors, such as high levels of poverty and community violence, predict high rates of aggression.[19] At more proximal levels, various parent-child interaction patterns are linked to aggression.[20,21] In particular, patterns characterised as highly coercive and lacking in emotional support and supervision predict aggression, both concurrently and in the future.[21] There has been some debate on the mechanism through which such factors contribute to aggression. Regardless of the precise mechanism, parent-child interactions are thought to be at least partially causally related to paediatric aggression, based on the replicated therapeutic effects of interventions designed to address poor parenting behaviours.[22] Nevertheless, parental factors represent only one cause of paediatric aggression.

Biological research also focuses on various levels of risk, from genetic to neuroanatomic factors. From the genetic perspective, family studies document considerable concordance between parental and child aggression.[23] Twin studies provide somewhat inconsistent data on the genetic contribution to such familial profiles, though more genetic studies examine patterns of delinquency than aggression. For ADHD, the data clearly suggest a role for genetic influences, with some recent data implicating specific dopamine-related genes.[24,25] The data for paediatric aggression, however, are less consistent than for ADHD.

From the perspective of brain systems, most research focuses on autonomic, neuropsychologicalal, or neurochemical aspects of aggression.[26-28] Autonomic signs of 'underarousal' relate to paediatric aggression, with the association between low resting heart rate and aggression representing the most robust biological finding in this area.[28] Other indices of low arousal include abnormal skin conductance and reduced levels of cortisol.[26-28] Indices of low arousal may particularly characterise chronically as opposed to transiently aggressive individuals.[29] Neuropsychological studies implicate the prefrontal or anterior temporal cortex in impulsive or aggressive behaviour, as manifested by either a frontal inhibitory deficit or a language-related temporal deficit.[7,30,31] From the neurochemical perspective, most research examines the role of catecholamines or indoleamines. As reviewed by others,[26,32,33] results in this area remain somewhat less consistent than in the areas of autonomic or neuropsychological measures.

The most recent research on ogy emphasises the interplay between biological and socio-environmental factors. One set of studies has relied on relatively large epidemiological samples to explore this issue. These studies have provided generalisable data but have relied on relatively crude biological indices. Another set of studies has relied on more precise biological indices, and has produced less generalisable conclusions. A detailed discussion of each study in this area is beyond the scope of this review, but the data clearly support a few key generalisations.

Epidemiological studies show that the interplay between biological and social or environmental factors predicts aggression better than the impact of either factor alone. Raine et al.[34] showed that children with perinatal complications faced a high risk for later violent behaviour when they were raised in a socially adverse environment, findings echoed in the data of Breslau.[35] Similarly, Pine et al.[36] found that minor physical anomalies, putative markers of abnormal brain development, increased the strength of the relationship between social risk factors and CD.

Studies of physiological systems suggest that family and environmental factors may affect the relationship between biology and behaviour. In studies of the serotonin (5-hydroxytryptamine; 5-HT) system, Pine et al.[32,37] found that parent-child interaction patterns related to markers of serotonergic function in children. These and other studies suggest that the relationship between serotonergic markers and aggression might vary as a function of environmental factors.[38,39] Raine et al.[40] generated similar findings in a positron emission tomography study of convicted murderers. Abnormalities in cerebral glucose metabolic rates were only found among murderers raised in the absence of adverse childhood social circumstances. These data are consistent with data on autonomic under-arousal, where the association between low arousal and aggression appears to be moderated by social adversity.[41,42]

In summary, paediatric aggression is a multidetermined phenomenon, even if relatively narrow behavioural constructs such as lifelong persistent aggression are considered. The most current research suggests that biological and socio-environmental factors both contribute to pathological aggression. Such research is consistent with data from treatment studies of the efficacy of psychotherapeutic and pharmacological interventions.

3. Therapeutics of Aggression

Although the current review emphasises pharmacology, given current data on ogical factors, pharmacology is likely to have more robust effects when used in the context of a broader intervention. We will not review data from psychotherapy studies on paediatric aggression, but the reader is referred to two recent reviews on the topic, one in patients with ADHD[43] and the other in patients with CD.[22]

Existing data suggest a role for psychotherapy in treating paediatric aggression, though data for ADHD are less conclusive. In fact, Hinshaw et al.[43] suggest that the role for psychotherapy remains unclear in ADHD uncomplicated by aggression. For aggression, Kazdin[22] suggests that extensive data support the beneficial effects of parent training and problem solving skills training techniques. While the data for other psychotherapies are limited, family-based treatments also show considerable promise.

In summarising the pharmacological approach to paediatric aggression, we first provide general guidelines for evaluating the existing research literature. As there is a growing emphasis on pharmacological research with children, these guidelines should prove helpful in evaluating future studies. We then provide brief summaries of the existing data for the most commonly prescribed treatments.

Conclusions on the efficacy of medications must be supported by treatment studies following standard guidelines, 4 of which we emphasise. First, given the episodic nature of paediatric aggression, conclusions on efficacy must follow from double-blind controlled studies, using random assignment to one of two medication conditions. Without such a design, any change in aggression following treatment might result either from day-to-day variability or from the effects of psychotherapeutic interventions, which are almost invariably part of any therapeutic encounter with children. Second, given the potential for psychotherapeutic effects, each medication should be compared against placebo. Third, the assessments should rely on multiple informants, including parents, the children themselves and teachers.

Some of the more frequently used scales, such as the Conners scales, appear in many of the studies summarised in table I. We review the existing literature on medication treatments for paediatric aggression, selecting studies that follow these three guidelines. These data are summarised in table I and in discussion presented below. Finally, in evaluating data from efficacy trials, it is important to consider both hypothesis testing and effect sizes. Data are most convincing when they show a statistical difference as well as a medium to large effect size. For the current review, we present effect sizes in table I, using the standardised difference score.[64] On this measure, a value of 0.5 is considered medium while a value of 0.8 and beyond is considered large. While the current review focuses on pharmacology, few of the studies in table I demonstrate large effects of pharmacological agents on aggression. As a result, it is important to consider other potential treatments for paediatric aggression.

3.1 Psychostimulants

Most studies examining the effect of psychostimulants in paediatric aggression involve children with ADHD. While there are 4 frequently used stimulants, only dexamphetamine and methylphenidate have been used in studies on paediatric aggression. As shown in table I, we located eight published randomised clinical trials using psychostimulants to treat children with ADHD complicated by high rates of aggression.[6,12,44-49] These trials either selected children with ADHD complicated by high ratings on a standardised aggression scale or selected children with ADHD complicated by another disruptive disorder. The results across these trials consistently show a strong beneficial effect of psychostimulants on paediatric aggression occurring in the context of ADHD.

There has been debate on the specificity for children with ADHD of the effect of psychostimulants on inattentiveness. This debate was largely resolved by Rapoport et al.[65] who showed that children without ADHD exhibit improvements in attention, much like children with ADHD, during stimulant treatment. A similar debate has arisen concerning the effects of psychostimulants on aggression. Until recently, psychostimulants were considered a good treatment for aggression primarily when associated with ADHD. However, Klein et al.[6] reported that methylphenidate was effective in treating aggression among children with CD, irrespective of ADHD symptomatology. While this suggests the utility of psychostimulants in treating CD, many of the children in this study had prior if not current histories of ADHD. Hence, the debate on the utility of psychostimulants in 'pure' CD or ODD is likely to persist.

It is important to note the advantages and risks associated with the use of psychostimulants. On the positive side, these medications have been well tolerated by children for more than 20

Table I. Randomised controlled trials of medications for paediatric aggression

Study	Gender	Sample (n)	Diagnosis (n)	Drug	Dosage	Measurement of response	Findings	Cohen's Standardised Difference Score (D)[a] [range]
Stimulants								
Klein et al.[6]	M/F	Outpatients (84)	CD with and without ADHD	Methylphenidate	60 mg/day maximum	Classroom observations, mood scales, achievement tests	Antisocial behaviours specific to CD were significantly reduced in drug group even when controlled for ADHD	Conduct problems: 1.67; aggression: 0.77
Hinshaw et al.[44]	M	Outpatients (22)	Comorbid ODD (10); CD (4)	Methylphenidate	7.5-15 mg/day	Laboratory setting. Group task with opportunity to cheat and steal	Decrease in stealing and property destruction; increase in cheating	NR
Gadow et al.[45]	M	Public classroom (11)	Aggressive/ hyperactive	Methylphenidate	0.3 and 0.6 mg/kg/day	Observed aggression directed at peers during structured and free play periods in classroom, lunchroom and recess	Drug did suppress observable aggression in natural environment, with best response in higher dose range; significant reduction of hyperactivity ratings	Range for placebo vs 0.3mg was 0.3-1.1; [placebo vs 0.6mg 0.4-1.1]
Arnold et al.[46]	NR	Outpatients (11)	Hyperkinetic and aggressive	Dexamphetamine Levoamphetamine	Mean 39 mg/day Mean 28.5-48 mg/day	Rating by psychiatrist, parent and teachers	Aggressive hostile behaviour is helped by both drugs, but anxiety and overactivity are helped more by dexamphetamine Significant drug effect	NR
Arnold et al.[47]	M/F	Outpatients (31)	Minimal brain dysfunction	Dexamphetamine Levoamphetamine	10-30 mg/day 14-49 mg/day	Behaviour checklists by teachers and parents	No significant drug effect	[placebo vs drug 0.2-0.7]
Conners et al.[12]	M	Inpatients (43)	Aggressive	Methylphenidate	20 mg/day	Symptom checklist, school reports, daily reports, Rosenzweig Picture Frustration Test; interview	No significant drug effect	NR
Kaplan et al.[48]	M	Inpatients (6)	Comorbid ADHD and aggressive CD	Methylphenidate	0.36-0.56 mg/kg/day	Measured aggressiveness with the Adolescent Anti-social Behaviour Checklist	Reduced verbal and physical aggressive symptoms	[0.6-0.9]
Pelham et al.[49]	M	Outpatients: prepubescent boys (17); adolescent boys (17)	ADHD	Methylphenidate	0.3 mg/kg/day	Daily counsellor behaviour observations	50% positive response rate. Did not specifically target aggression	[0.27-0.35]
Clonidine								
Jaselskis et al.[50]	M	Outpatients (8)	Autistic, excess hyperactivity, inattention, impulsivity. Not tolerating other medication	Clonidine	0.15-0.2 mg/day; 3 times a day	Teacher ratings on aberrant behaviour, checklist, Conners Parent-Teacher Questionnaire	33% decrease in irritability. Teacher and parent ratings decreased with drug use	[0.34-0.67]

Reference	Sex	Patients (n)	Diagnosis	Drug	Dose	Assessment measures	Results	Effect size
Hunt et al.[51]	M	Outpatients (10)	ADHD	Clonidine	4-5 µg/kg/day maximum	Conners Parent-Teacher Questionnaire, Kagan Matching Familiar Figures, clinicians blind global ratings	Drug significantly improved overall behaviour ratings of impulsivity, hyperactivity and inattention	[0.9-1.4]
Antipsychotics								
Cunningham et al.[52]	M/F	Inpatients (12)	Aggressive, hyperactive, nonpsychotic	Haloperidol	3 mg/day	Behaviour checklist - ward and school	8/12 children were rated as generally improved in the ward; no significant difference in school behaviour	NR
Werry & Aman[53]	M	Outpatients (24)	Hyperkinetic and unsocialised aggressive; nonpsychotic	Haloperidol	0.25 mg/kg/day; 0.05 mg/kg/day	Attention, immediate recognition, memory, reaction times and seat activity	No significant drug effect	NR
Campbell et al.[54]	M/F	Inpatients (61)	Aggressive CD; adolescents previously resistant to treatment	Haloperidol Lithium	1-16 mg/day 500-2000 mg/day	Children's Psychiatric Rating Scale; Clinical Global Impression	Efficacy of 2 drugs equivalent, but superior to placebo	NR
Greenhill et al.[55]	M/F	Inpatients (31)	Undersocialised CD; aggressive type	Molindone Thioridazine	2.5-10 mg/kg/day 0.5-2 mg/kg/day	Conner's Rating Scale, Conner's Teacher Questionnaire, Children's Psychiatric Rating Scale, Inpatient Aggression Scales, Clinical Global Impression	Both drugs produced significant decrease in hostility, antisocial and violence subscales	NR
Campbell et al.[56]	M/F	Inpatients (10)	Schizophrenia (7); 'behaviour disordered' (2); 'organic brain disorder' (1)	Combined lithium and chlorpromazine	Chlorpromazine 15-90 mg/day; lithium 450-1350 mg/day	Clinical Global Impression, symptom checklist	Only 1 child showed marked improvement in aggressiveness	NR
Lithium								
Campbell et al.[56]	M/F	Inpatients (10)	Schizophrenia (7); 'behaviour disordered' (2); 'organic brain disorder' (1)	Combined lithium and chlorpromazine	Chlorpromazine 15-90 mg/day; lithium 450-1350 mg/day	Clinical Global Impression, symptom checklist	Only 1 child showed marked improvement in aggressiveness	NR
Campbell et al.[54]	M/F	Inpatients (61)	Aggressive CD; adolescents previously resistant to treatment	Haloperidol Lithium	1-16 mg/day 500-2000 mg/day	Children's Psychiatric Rating Scale and Clinical Global Impression	Efficacy of 2 drugs equivalent, but superior to placebo	NR

Continued over page

Table I. Contd

Study	Gender	Sample (n)	Diagnosis (n)	Drug	Dosage	Measurement of response	Findings	Cohen's Standardised Difference Score (D)[a]
Sheard et al.[57]	M	Prisoners (66)	Nonpsychotic	Lithium	Maintain serum lithium concentrations of 0.6-1 mmol/L	Infractions in jail, behaviour rating scales, Lykken Sociopathy Scale, projective and personality tests	Drug group had significantly fewer infractions	NR
Rifkin et al.[58]	M/F	Inpatients (33)	CD	Lithium	600 mg/day; maintain blood concentrations of 0.6-1.0 mmol/L	Behaviour rating scale, Hamilton Rating Scale for Depression, Side Effect Scale, ADHD Adolescent Self Report, Conner's Teacher Rating Scale	No significant drug effect	NR
Malone et al.[59]	M/F	Inpatients (24)	CD	Lithium	NR	Aggression questionnaire	Treatment response was associated with a 'more affective' type of aggression	NR
Campbell et al.[60]	M/F	Inpatients (50)	CD	Lithium	600-2100 mg/day	Conners' Parent-Teacher Questionnaire, Global Clinical Judgements Scale, Children's Psychiatric Rating Scale, Conner's Teacher Questionnaire, POMS-self report	Significant drug effect	NR
Anticonvulsants								
Lefkowitz[61]	M	Inpatients (50)	Aggressive, disruptive	Phenytoin	200 mg/day	Psychopathology, personality, mood, behaviour scales	No significant effect. Placebo group were less aggressive at end of trial	NR
Looker & Conners[62]	M/F	Outpatients (17)	Aggressive, assaultive	Phenytoin	100-200 mg/day	Parent/school symptom checklist, cognitive tests	Parent/school ratings showed no significant drug effect	NR
Conners et al.[12]	M	Inpatients (43)	Aggressive	Phenytoin	200 mg/day	Symptom checklist, school reports, daily reports, Rosenzweig Picture Frustration test, interview	No significant drug effect	NR
Cueva et al.[63]	M/F	Outpatients (22)	CD	Carbamazepine	400-800 mg/day	Rating scales	No significant drug effect	NR

a   Scores increase with increased effect.[64]

ADHD = attention deficit hyperactivity disorder; **CD** = conduct disorder; **F** = female; **M** = male; **n** = number of patients; **NR** = not recorded; **ODD** = oppositional defiant disorder; **POMS** = Profile of Mood States.

years. Adverse effects are generally mild, though clinicians should alert patients and families to the potential adverse effects, including changes in mood or anxiety, decreased appetite, headache and gastrointestinal complaints. Other adverse effects that should be discussed include growth suppression and exacerbation of tics. While psychostimulants can suppress growth, this can be avoided through medication 'holidays' whereupon the medication is discontinued during school vacations. Lowering the medication dose may also have a beneficial effect. Similarly, psychostimulants can exacerbate tics in some children, but the most recent research suggests that the medications are well tolerated in many children with tics.[66,67] When tics are exacerbated by stimulants, the exacerbations may be only mild, and the benefits in terms of controlling other symptoms may outweigh the risks associated with tic exacerbation.

Finally, clinicians should note the abuse potential of psychostimulants, particularly in chronically aggressive children who face a high risk for substance abuse (ric aggression is a strong risk factor for substance abuse). Again, while there is minimal evidence that psycho-stimulants contribute to the development of substance abuse, children who are already showing signs of such behaviour may inappropriately use these medications. There has been some suggestion that pemoline is less likely to be abused than other stimulant medications, but enthusiasm for this medication has been tempered by reports of hepatotoxicity.

3.2 Lithium

After psychostimulants, lithium remains perhaps the most extensively studied medication for treating aggression in children with disruptive disorders. As shown in table I, six studies were identified.[54,56-60] The data from these studies are mixed. Campbell et al.[54] initially reported a moderate positive effect on aggression among psychiatric inpatients, but a sub-sequent follow-up study reported weaker, though still significant, effects.[60] Malone et al.[59] also reported relatively strong positive effects. Rifkin et al.,[58] in contrast, found virtually no effect of lithium in CD. Hence, firm conclusions on efficacy await the results of subsequent trials. In light of recent studies emphasising the potentially strong relationships among ADHD, bipolar disorder and aggression, more randomised controlled trials appear indicated, particu-larly in children with signs of ADHD, mania and aggressive behaviour.[3] Of note, prior open trials of lithium for the treatment of ADHD find little evidence of efficacy, though these trials did not select ADHD children with either signs of aggression or mania. A recent, controlled trial suggests that lithium is in fact beneficial for adolescent mania.[68]

The use of lithium is complicated by the relatively narrow 'therapeutic window' of the medication, such that there is a relatively small difference between therapeutic and toxic doses of the medication. Even when prescribed in appropriate dosages, a number of effects can be troublesome to children, including effects on arousal level, cognition, motor function and urinary frequency. These adverse effects are generally dose related. On the other hand, Campbell et al.[54] suggested that the adverse effects are better tolerated than those that occur with antipsychotics. Moreover, the adverse effects are completely reversible, unlike the poten-tial neurological adverse effects of antipsychotics. Given the fact that there are some data that suggest lithium is effective, this medication is a reasonable treatment for families who can monitor the use of the medication appropriately.

3.3 Antipsychotics

Table I presents data from five studies examining the efficacy of antipsychotics in aggression.[52-56] Across the studies, various agents have been shown to effectively reduce aggression. As a result, there is some justification for the frequent use of these medications in chronically aggressive children. Of note, there are no data on the utility of the newer atypical antipsychotics in paediatric aggression. These newer agents may pose less risk of severe neurological sequelae. Studies in the US are currently examining the efficacy of atypical antipsychotics in CD.

The risk of tardive dyskinesia remains a major limitation with antipsychotics. While caution is urged when using antipsychotics in any child, particular care seems warranted in disruptive disorders. Given the chronic nature of aggression in disruptive disorders, children treated with antipsychotics are at risk of long term exposure. Accordingly, antipsychotic drugs should only be used sparingly in aggressive children and only after other medications have failed to control severely problematic behaviour. Beyond their neurological adverse effects, antipsychotics possess a number of other adverse effects. Campbell et al.[54] suggest that the cognitive effects may be particularly troublesome, though the risk for dystonia and anticholinergic effects should also be kept in mind.

3.4 Anticonvulsants

There has been a long-standing interest in the use of anticonvulsants to treat paediatric aggression. Initially, this interest was fuelled by reports of an association between epilepsy and violence in children.[69] More recently, there has been considerable interest in the potential associations among bipolar disorder, seizure activity and aggressive behaviour.[70] A number of anticonvulsants, including carbamazepine and valproic acid (sodium valproate), are beneficial in adult bipolar disorder, reducing irritable aggression associated with some forms of mixed manic states. Furthermore, anticonvulsants may reduce aggressive behaviour among children with overt epilepsy. The use of anticonvulsants in these scenarios, however, should be distinguished from the use in other clinical scenarios.

Of most relevance for the current review, there are minimal data supporting the efficacy of anticonvulsants in disruptive behaviour disorders. As shown in table I, the only randomised controlled trial of carbamazepine found little evidence of efficacy[63] while earlier trials of phenytoin, as shown in table I, were similarly unimpressive.[12,61,62] While there are data from open trials of other anticonvulsant medications that suggest a possible role in paediatric aggression, definitive conclusions on efficacy must await data from randomised controlled trials.

Given the limited data on efficacy, the adverse effects of the anticonvulsants will only be briefly mentioned. Each anticonvulsant used to treat paediatric aggression has been linked to potentially serious adverse effects. For carbamazepine, these include effects on the tological and cardiovascular system. For valproic acid, these include effects on the hepatic and genito-urinary systems, at least in female participants. When combined with the limited data on efficacy, the adverse effects associated with each of these medications limit their use in paediatric aggression.

3.5 α_2-Agonists

As with the anticonvulsants, interest in the use of α_2-agonists arises more from theoretic considerations than data in clinical trials. Two such medications, clonidine and guanfacine, have been used. These medications reduce firing of the locus ceruleus, and earlier theories suggested that this effect might decrease certain forms of aggression associated with increased noradrenergic outflow.[51] On the other hand, medications with stimulatory effects on the noradrenergic system, including stimulants and carbamazepine, are used to treat aggression. As a result, more recent theories on α_2-agonists emphasise effects at postsynaptic receptors in the prefrontal cortex, whereby the medications might either increase attention or inhibitory control by activating relevant circuits.[71] Despite such theoretic support, only two clinical trials have examined the effects of these medications on aggression.

Hunt et al.[51] found evidence of a positive effect of clonidine in a small trial, while Jaselskis et al.[50] also found evidence for a beneficial effect of clonidine in a trial for children with pervasive developmental disorders. No controlled data are available for guanfacine, though suggestive data emerge in open trials. These data have been criticised from various perspectives,[72] and the agents are not considered first-line treatments for paediatric aggression. Critics emphasise the risk of cardiovascular incidents with the medications, as well as the limited data on efficacy.[72]

3.6 Other Agents

While research reviewed above provides the most complete data on the efficacy of pharmacological treatments for aggression, other agents are frequently used as well. Such agents include serotonergic medications, β-blockers and combination approaches. In contrast to research reviewed in sections 3.1 to 3.5, limited conclusions can be drawn for these other agents because of the lack of data from randomised controlled trials. Nevertheless, the available data will be briefly discussed.

Data to support the use of serotonergic medications derive from studies in adults. A wealth of research clearly links serotonergic indices to indices of aggression among adults, particularly when aggression is impulsive or emotive in nature. Fluoxetine, a selective serotonin reuptake inhibitor, has been successfully trialled in adults with aggression accompanying personality disorders.[73] Medications, such as the azapirones, with agonist effects on the serotonin 5-HT_{1A} receptor have also been proposed as a treatment for adult aggression. However, there are insufficient data from clinical trials to fully support their use in adults. While the data are sparse in adults, they are virtually nonexistent in children. A few open studies suggest relatively modest effects of either selective serotonin reuptake inhibitors or 5-HT_{1A} agonists in paediatric aggression. However, the medications should not be considered first-line treatments for aggression, as no data from randomised clinical trials are available.

Data among adults also suggest a role for β-blockers in the treatment of aggression, particularly when it accompanies organic mental syndromes.[13,74] Typically, very high levels of medication have been used, and the relevance of such interventions for children with disruptive behaviour disorders remains unclear.

Finally, since chronic aggression in the context of a disruptive disorder is often treatment refractory, a number of combination approaches have been used. Safer[75] noted the increasing reliance on such 'polypharmaceutical' treatments in children. Given the lack of data on efficacy, let alone evidence of tolerability, such combination treatments should be used with caution. For example, there was initial enthusiasm for combining stimulants with α_2-agonists in the treatment of behaviour disorders, but concerns have been raised on the tolerability of such combinations.[72]

4. Conclusions

This review is focused on aggression that arises as part of the disruptive behaviour disorders, since this form of aggression is most commonly confronted in clinics and is associated with high levels of impairment. Results from studies suggest the availability of various treatments for reducing paediatric aggression. Nevertheless, there is wide variation in the magnitude of effect of the available treatments, with most studies showing relatively modest effects. Hence, even when treatments are successful, aggressive behaviour tends to be reduced, but generally fails to reach normal levels. As a result, therapeutic approaches that combine pharmaco-therapies with other modalities are likely to be necessary in the management of many children but should be used with caution.

Acknowledgements

Dr Pine and Ms Cohen are supported by NIMH Center Grant MH-43878 to the Center to Study Youth Anxiety, Suicide, and Depression. A Scientist Development Award for Clinicians from NIMH was awarded to Dr Pine (K20-MH01391).

References

1. Achenbach TM, McConaughy SH, Howell CT. Child/adolescent behavioral and emotional problems: implications of cross-informant correlations for situational specificity. Psychol Bull 1987; 101: 213-32
2. Cantwell D, Rutter M. Classification: conceptual issues and substantive findings. In: Rutter M, Taylor E, Hersov L, editors. Child and adolescent psychiatry: modern approaches. Oxford: Blackwell Scientific Publications, 1994: 3-21
3. Wozniak J, Biederman J. A pharmacological approach to the quagmire of comorbidity in juvenile mania. J Am Acad Child Adolesc Psychiatry 1996; 35: 826-8
4. Moffitt TE. Adolescence-limited and life-course-persistent antisocial behavior: a developmental taxonomy. Psychol Rev 1993; 100: 674-701
5. Hinshaw SP, Heller T, McHale JP. Covert antisocial behavior in boys with attention-deficit hyperactivity disorder: external validation and effects of methylphenidate. J Consult Clin Psychol 1992; 60: 274-81
6. Klein RG, Abikoff H, Klass E, et al. Clinical efficacy of methylphenidate in conduct disorder with and without attention deficit hyperactivity disorder. Arch Gen Psychiatry 1997; 54: 1073-80
7. Oosterlaan J. Response inhibition in children with attention deficit hyperactivity and related disorders. New York: Plenum Publishing Corporation, 1996
8. Taylor E. Syndromes of attention deficit and overactivity. In: Rutter M, Taylor E, Hersov L, editors. Child and adolescent psychiatry: modern approaches. Oxford: Blackwell Scientific Publications, 1994: 285-307
9. Earls F. Oppositional–defiant and conduct disorders. In: Rutter M, Taylor E, Hersov L, editors. Child and adolescent psychiatry: modern approaches. Oxford: Blackwell Scientific Publications, 1994: 308-29
10. Mannuzza S, Klein RG, Konig PH, et al. Childhood predictors of psychiatric status in the young adulthood of hyperactive boys: a study controlling for chance association. In: Robins L, Rutter M, editors. Straight and devious pathways from childhood to adulthood. New York: Cambridge University Press, 1990: 279-99
11. Vitiello B, Stoff DM. Subtypes of aggression and their relevance to child psychiatry. J Am Acad Child Adolesc Psychiatry 1997; 36: 307-15
12. Conners CK, Kramer R, Rothschild G, et al. Treatment of young delinquent boys with diphenylhydantoin sodium and methyphenidate: a controlled comparison. Arch Gen Psychiatry 1971; 24: 156-60
13. Yudofsky SC, Silver JM, Jackson W, et al. The Overt Aggression Scale for the objective rating of verbal and physical aggression. Am J Psychiatry 1986; 143: 35-9
14. Olweus D. Stability of aggressive reaction patterns in males: a review. Psychol Bull 1979; 86: 852-75
15. Huesmann LR, Eron LD, Yarmel PW. Intellectual functioning and aggression. J Pers Soc Psychol 1987; 52: 232-40
16. Robins LN. Sturdy childhood predictors of adult antisocial behaviour: replications from longitudinal studies. Psychol Med 1978; 8: 611-22
17. Farrington D, Loeber R, Van Kammen WB. Long-term criminal outcomes of hyperactivity-impulsivity-attention deficit and conduct problems in childhood. In: Robins L, Rutter M, editors. Straight and devious pathways from childhood to adulthood. New York: Cambridge University Press, 1990: 279-99
18. Rutter M, Giller H. Juvenile delinquency: trends and perspectives. New York: Guilford Press, 1983
19. Sampson RJ, Raudenbush SW, Earls F. Neighborhoods and violent crime: a multilevel study of collective efficacy. Science 1997; 277: 918-24
20. Dodge KA, Bates JE, Pettit GS. Mechanisms in the cycle of violence. Science 1990; 250: 1678-83
21. Wasserman GA, Miller LS, Pinner E, et al. Parenting predictors of early conduct problems in urban, high-risk boys. J Am Acad Child Adolesc Psychiatry 1996; 35: 1227-36

22. Kazdin AE. Psychosocial treatments for conduct disorder in children. In: Nathan P, Gorman J, editors. A guide to treatments that work. New York: Oxford University Press, 1998: 65-89
23. Cadoret RJ, Yates WR, Troughton E, et al. Genetic-environmental interaction in the genesis of aggressivity and conduct disorders. Arch Gen Psychiatry 1995; 52: 916-24
24. Cook Jr EH, Stein MA, Krasowski MD, et al. Association of attention-deficit disorder and the dopamine transporter gene. Am J Hum Genet 1995; 56 (4): 993-8
25. LaHoste GJ, Swanson JM, Wigal SB, et al. Dopamine D4 receptor gene polymorphism is associated with attention deficit hyperactivity disorder. Mol Psychiatry 1996; 1: 83-4
26. McBurnett K, Lahey BB, Capasso L, et al. Aggressive symptoms and salivary cortisol in clinic-referred boys with conduct disorder. Ann N Y Acad Sci 1996; 794: 169-78
27. Raine A, Brennan P, Mednick B, et al. High rates of violence, crime, academic problems, and behavioral problems in males with both early neuromotor deficits and unstable family environments. Arch Gen Psychiatry 1996; 53: 544-9
28. Raine A. The psychopathology of crime: criminal behavior as a clinical disorder. San Diego: Academic Press Inc., 1993
29. Raine A, Venables PH, Williams M. Relationships between central and autonomic measures of arousal at age 15 years and criminality at age 24 years. Arch Gen Psychiatry 1990; 47: 1003-7
30. Pennington BF, Ozonoff S. Executive functions and developmental psychopathology. J Child Psychol Psychiatry 1996; 37: 51-87
31. Pine DS, Bruder GE, Wasserman GA, et al. Verbal dichotic listening in boys at risk for behavior disorders. J Am Acad Child Adolesc Psychiatry 1997; 36: 1465-73
32. Pine DS, Coplan JD, Wasserman G, et al. Neuroendocrine response to fenfluramine challenge in boys: associations with aggressive behavior and adverse rearing. Arch Gen Psychiatry 1997; 54 (9): 785-9
33. Rogeness GA, Javors MA, Pliszka SR. Neurochemistry and child and adolescent psychiatry. J Am Acad Child Adolesc Psychiatry 1992; 31: 765-81
34. Raine A, Brennan P, Mednick SA. Birth complications combined with early maternal rejection at age 1 year predispose to violent crime at age 18 years. Arch Gen Psychiatry 1994; 51: 984-8
35. Breslau N. Psychiatric sequelae of low birth weight. Epidemiol Rev 1995; 17: 96-104
36. Pine DS, Shaffer D, Schonfeld IS, et al. Minor physical anomalies: modifiers of environmental risks for psychiatric impairment. J Am Acad Child Adolesc Psychiatry 1997; 36: 395-403
37. Pine DS, Wasserman G, Coplan J, et al. Associations between platelet serotonin-2A receptor characteristics and parenting factors in boys at risk for delinquency. Am J Psychiatry 1996; 153: 538-44
38. Halperin JM, Newcorn JH, Kopstein I, et al. Serotonin, aggression, and parental psychopathology in children with attention-deficit hyperactivity disorder. J Am Acad Child Adolesc Psychiatry 1997; 36: 1391-8
39. Kruesi MJ, Hibbs ED, Zahn TP, et al. A 2-year prospective follow-up study of children and adolescents with disruptive behavior disorders: prediction by cerebrospinal fluid 5-hydroxyindoleacetic acid, homovanillic acid, and autonomic measures? Arch Gen Psychiatry 1992; 49: 429-35
40. Raine A, Stoddard J, Bihrle S, et al. Prefrontal glucose deficits in murderers lacking psychosocial deprivation. Neuropsychiatry Neuropsychol Behav Neurol 1997; 42: 495-508
41. Raine A, Venables PH. Tonic heart rate level, social class and antisocial behaviour in adolescents. Biol Psychol 1984; 18: 123-32
42. Wadsworth MEJ. Delinquency, pulse rate and early emotional deprivation. Br J Criminol 1976; 16: 245-56
43. Hinshaw SP, Klein RG, Abikoff H. Childhood attention deficit hyperactivity disorder: nonpharmacological and combination treatments. In: Nathan P, Gorman J, editors. A guide to treatments that work. New York: Oxford University Press, 1998: 26-41
44. Hinshaw SP, Heller T, McHale JP. Covert antisocial behavior in boys with attention-deficit hyperactivity disorder: external validation and effects of methylphenidate. J Consult Clin Psychol 1992; 60: 274-81
45. Gadow KD, Nolan EE, Sverd J, et al. Methylphenidate in aggressive-hyperactive boys: I: effects on peer aggression in public school settings. J Am Acad Child Adolesc Psychiatry 1990; 29; 710-8
46. Arnold LE, Kirilcuk V, Corson SA, et al. Levoamphetamine and dextroamphetamine: differential effect on aggression and hyperkenisis in children and dogs. Am J Psychiatry 1973; 130: 165-70
47. Arnold LE, Huestis RD, Smeltzer DJ, et al. Levoamphetamine vs dextroamphetamine in minimal brain dysfunction: replication, time response, and differential effect by diagnostic group and family rating. Arch Gen Psychiatry 1976; 33: 292-301
48. Kaplan S, Busner J, Kupietz S, et al. Effects of methylphenidate on adolescents with aggressive conduct disorder and ADDH: a preliminary report. J Am Acad Child Adolesc Psychiatry 1990; 29: 719-23
49. Pelham WE, Vodde-Hamilton M, Murphy D, et al. The effects of methylphenidate on ADHD adolescents in recreational, peer group, and classroom setting. J Clin Child Psychol 1991; 20: 293-300
50. Jaselskis CA, Cook EH, Fletcher KE, et al. Clonidine treatment of hyperactive and impulsive children with autistic disorder. J Clin Psychopharmacol 1992: 12: 322-7
51. Hunt RD, Ruud MB, Cohen DJ. The therapeutic effect of clonidine in attention deficit disorder with hyperactivity: a comparison with placebo and methylphenidate. Psychopharmacol Bull 1986; 22: 229-36
52. Cunningham MA, Pillai V, Rogers WJB. Halperidol in the treatment of children with severe behaviour disorders. Br J Psychiatry 1968; 114: 845-54
53. Werry JS, Aman MG. Methylphenidate and haloperidol in children: effects on attention, memory, and activity. Arch Gen Psychiatry 1975; 327: 90-5

54. Campbell M, Small A, Green W, et al. Behavioral efficacy of haloperidol and lithium carbonate: a comparison in hospitalized aggressive children with conduct disorder. Arch Gen Psychiatry 1984; 41: 650-6
55. Greenhill L, Solomon M, Pleak R, et al. Molindone hydrochloride treatment of hospitalized children with conduct disorder. J Clin Psychiatry 1985; 46: 20-5
56. Campbell M, Fish B, Korein J, et al. Lithium and chlorpromazine: a controlled crossover study of hyperactive severely disturbed young children. J Autism Child Schizophrenia 1972; 2: 234-63
57. Sheard MH, Marini JL, Bridges CI, et al. The effect of lithium on impulsive aggressive behavior in man. Am J Psychiatry 1976; 133: 1409-13
58. Rifkin A, Karajgi B, Dicker R, et al. Lithium treatment of conduct disorders in adolescents. Am J Psychiatry 1997; 154: 554-5
59. Malone RP, Bennet DS, Luebbert JF, et al. Aggression classification and treatment response. Psychopharmacol Bull 1998; 34 (1): 41-5
60. Campbell M, Adams PB, Small AM, et al. Lithium in hospitalized aggressive children with conduct disorder: a double-blind and placebo-controlled study. J Am Acad Child Adolesc Psychiatry 1995; 34: 445-53
61. Lefkowitz MM. Effects of diphenylhydantoin on disruptive behavior. Arch Gen Psychiatry 1969; 20: 643-51
62. Looker A, Conners CK. Diphenylhydantoin in children with severe temper tantrums. Arch Gen Psychiatry 1970; 23: 80-9
63. Cueva JE, Overall J, Small A, et al. Carbamazepine in aggressive children with conduct disorder: a double-blind and placebo-controlled study. J Am Acad Child Adolesc Psychiatry 1996; 35: 480-90
64. Cohen J. Statistical power for the behavioral sciences. Rev. ed. Hillsdale (NJ): Lawrence Erlbaum, 1987
65. Rapoport JL, Buchsbaum MS, Zahn TP, et al. Dextroamphetamine: cognitive and behavioral effects in normal prepubertal boys. Science 1978; 199: 560-3
66. Castellanos FX, Giedd JN, Elia J, et al. Controlled stimulant treatment of ADHD and comorbid Tourette's syndrome: effects of stimulant and dose. J Am Acad Child Adolesc Psychiatry 1997; 36: 589-96
67. Gadow KD, Sverd J, Sprafkin J, et al. Efficacy of methylphenidate for attention-deficit hyperactivity disorder in children with tic disorder. Arch Gen Psychiatry 1995; 52: 444-55
68. Geller B, Cooper TB, Sun K, et al. Double-blind and placebo controlled study of lithium for adolescent bipolar disorders with secondary substance dependence. J Am Acad Child Adolesc Psychiatry 1998; 37: 171-8
69. Lewis DO, Pincus JH, Shanok SS, et al. Psychomotor epilepsy and violence in a group of incarcerated adolescent boys. Am J Psychiatry 1982; 139: 882-7
70. Post RM, Ketter TA, Denicoff K, et al. The place of anticonvulsant therapy in bipolar illness. Psychopharmacology 1996; 128: 115-29
71. Arnsten AF, Steere JC, Hunt RD. The contribution of alpha 2-noradrenergic mechanisms of prefrontal cortical cognitive function: potential significance for attention-deficit hyperactivity disorder. Arch Gen Psychiatry 1996; 53: 448-55
72. Cantwell DP, Swanson J, Connor DF. Case study: adverse response to clonidine. J Am Acad Child Adolesc Psychiatry 1997; 36: 39-44
73. Coccaro EF, Kavoussi RJ. Fluoxetine and impulsive aggressive behavior in personality disordered subjects. Arch Gen Psychiatry 1997; 54: 1081-8
74. Ratey JJ, Sorgi P, O'Driscoll GA, et al. Nadolol to treat aggression and psychiatric symptomatology in chronic psychiatric inpatients: a double-blind, placebo-controlled study. J Clin Psychiatry 1992; 53 (2): 41-6
75. Safer DJ. Changing patterns of psychotropic medications prescribed by child psychiatrists in the 1990s. J Child Adolesc Psychopharmacol 1997; 7: 267-74

Correspondence: Dr *Daniel S. Pine*, New York State Psychiatric Institute, Box 74, 1051 Riverside Drive, New York, NY 10032, USA.

Autism
Role of Drug Treatment and a Guide to its Use

Jan K. Buitelaar and *Erica M. Harteveld*

Department of Child Psychiatry, Academisch Ziekenhuis Utrecht, Utrecht,
The Netherlands

The aim of this review is to give a succinct overview of the diagnostic and therapeutic approaches to children, adolescents and adults with autism and other pervasive developmental disorders. Since Kanner[1] introduced the syndrome of early infantile autism into the psychiatric literature, the concept and definition of autism has been revised and adapted several times by both clinicians and researchers. The definition of autism has now been modified to become conceptually identical in the two commonly used classification systems, the International Classification of Diseases of the World Health Organization[2] and the DSM-IV of the American Psychiatric Association.[3] The key elements in both systems are: (i) severe and pervasive impairments in the development of social interaction and communication; (ii) unusual interests and stereotyped patterns of behaviour; and (iii) an onset prior to age 3 years.

It has become accepted that autism is a neurodevelopmental disorder with an heterogeneous atiology.[4] Although genetic influences are thought to play a major part, adverse prenatal and perinatal factors and concomitant medical disorders also seem to be important. Autism is associated with mental retardation in 65 to 90% of cases.[5]

In the DSM-IV, autism is classified as a pervasive developmental disorder. The term 'pervasive' is used to stress that the disorder concerns a group of children and adults with severe difficulties in social and communicative skills, other than problems caused by general developmental delay.[6] In addition to autism, a number of related conditions have been subsumed among the pervasive developmental disorders, such as Rett's disorder, childhood disintegrative disorder, Asperger's disorder and pervasive developmental disorder not otherwise specified (PDD-NOS). In this review, we use the term 'autism' to denote all the pervasive developmental disorders.

1. Diagnosis

Despite the very early onset of autism, children with suspected autism are rarely referred to a specialist centre before 3 years of age. This relatively late age of detection seems to be due to a combination of factors.[7] First, autism is a rare disorder, with a prevalence estimated at 10 to 20 cases per 10 000. Secondly, developmental screening routines in most countries focus on the screening of motor, intellectual and perceptual development, all of which may appear normal in children with autism. Thirdly, the diagnostic criteria include a number of social and communicative behaviours that emerge in the course of normal development from age 2.5 years onward. Therefore, it takes some time before it can be established that the child is not merely developing more slowly than is normal.

On referral, the diagnosis should be established after a comprehensive clinical assessment, which should include:
- a detailed developmental history
- an interview with the parents, with systematic probes for behavioural symptoms and peculiarities
- a semi-structured behavioural observation of the child
- psychological testing.

The assessment may include the use of standardised screening and diagnostic instruments[8] such as the Childhood Autistic Rating Scale,[9] the Autism Diagnostic Interview-Revised[10] and the Autism Diagnostic Observation Schedule.[11] The latter 2 instruments have been mainly developed for research purposes, and the interviewer must be trained in their use.

In about 10 to 37% of cases, autism is associated with specific medical disorders and/or organic conditions.[12] Although there is consensus that a thorough medical examination is needed, different centres of expertise have different opinions about the justifiability of the routine use of invasive procedures such as lumbar punctures and neuroimaging.[13] A more cautious approach is a standard medical history, meticulous physical examination, an EEG to rule out subclinical epilepsy, chromosomal culture and gene analysis, and blood and urine tests to detect metabolic disorders. High priority should also be given to a careful assessment of hearing and vision. This is important because sensory deficits may easily go undetected in individuals with autism and, moreover, may contribute to the emergence of autistic symptoms.

After the diagnostic process has been completed, it is essential to take time to share with the parents the information about the diagnosis and its implications for the further development of the child. Genetic counselling may also be necessary.

2. General Principles of Treatment

Autism is a chronically disabling condition for which no effective cure exists. The treatment of patients with autism should be multimodal, with a combination of structured and special educational techniques, individual behaviour modification, home training, family counselling, and placement in special schools or daycare centres. Drug treatment may benefit a number of patients, but should be given as a component of a comprehensive treatment approach.

In his outline of the principles of treatment of autism, Rutter[14] indicates that the main aim is to strive for normal development. He lists 4 areas from which goals for treatment must be derived:
- The facilitation and stimulation of the development of cognition, language and socialisation.
- The decreasing of autism-bound maladaptive behaviours such as rigidity, stereotypy and inflexibility.
- The elimination of nonspecific maladaptive behaviours such as hyperactivity and disruptive behaviour.
- The alleviation of family distress.

Different forms of treatment are available to achieve these goals.[6]

2.1 Family Support

It is essential to provide family support. When parents hear about autism for the first time, they are usually not fully aware that the upbringing of their child will be very difficult for themselves and his/her siblings. It is very important to inform the parents about the diagnosis and implications for the future of the child. Parents can have difficulty in accepting the diagnosis. The clinician must guide them to the available treatment facilities and coordinate the child's care. During the different stages of development, the child and the parents can have different needs. For example, placement in a school that provides specialised education can be enough for the first years, but when behaviour management problems occur, more intensive counselling, behavioural therapy and/or medication can be an option. It is crucial to help families find support systems that will help diminish their distress. National Autistic Societies in several countries hold, among other events, information evenings where parents can meet each other and where 'non-professional' support is given.

2.2 Education

Opportunities for adequate education are essential, as follow-up studies have indicated that children with autism who complete some form of education have a better outcome.[15] It is necessary for the teacher to be informed about the nature of autism and the child's needs. An autistic child at school needs extra individual attention, a very structured approach and special education programmes, such as the Treatment and Education of Autistic and Related Communication Handicapped Children programme (TEACCH, described by Campbell and Schopler[16]). This programme emphasises extensive collaboration with and training of the parents, so that they become knowledgable about their child's disorder and needs. This programme provides a highly structured approach for autistic children at school. Based on principles from cognitive and behavioural theory, a system is developed with step-by-step visualisation of the actions needed to fulfil a task. Through this system the life-environment can be structured, and parents can act as co-therapists and continue with the principles of TEACCH at home.

2.3 Skills Training and Behavioural Therapy

Depending on clinical needs, a number of specific treatment modalities may be helpful. In cases of clumsiness or delays in motor development, there is an indication for sensorimotor training. Language and communication skills may be facilitated by means of language training. Occupational and play therapy may be of use in some patients. For high functioning autistic children, individual therapy can be an option, when the child is, for instance, suffering from the awareness of being different. Social skills training programmes, delivered on an individual or group base, are increasingly being offered to children and adolescents with autism.[17,18] Recently, social skills training programmes have been nurtured using ideas from research on the theory of mind and emotional recognition deficits in autism. Although the benefits may be an improvement of social awareness and the acquisition of routine social skills, the long term benefits are often disappointing due to a lack of generalisation of skills.

Behavioural treatment based on classical and operant conditioning is the most studied and publicised form of nonmedical treatment for autism. There is a clear indication for specific behavioural interventions in individuals with severe maladaptive behaviours such as stereotypes, self-injury and negativism that interfere with their functioning. The acquisition of normal behaviours, such as toileting behaviours, may also benefit from behavioural interventions. These interventions should be based on a detailed analysis of the functional relationship between the child and the environment.[16] After the analysis, an individual treatment plan can be designed for the child. The child's behaviour is modified through techniques such as reinforcement by material or social rewards. Lovaas[19] described a long term behavioural intervention project with very intensive treatment in 19 young autistic children. He claimed that intensive behavioural treatment can significantly alter outcome. However, this promising result, and that of a related study,[20] have been questioned because of methodological problems.[21] In the Utrecht clinic for child psychiatry, we use elements derived from cognitive therapy in the treatment programmes of high functioning children who have pervasive developmental disorder. The central goal of therapy is to train the children to distinguish and order thoughts and feelings so that they can learn to cope with them and prevent emotional outbursts.

2.4 Vocational Training and Social Support

Autism is a life-long disorder that impacts on the ability of individuals to obtain employment, care for themselves and live independently. As a result, many individuals with autism require some sort of community support. Vocational training and support allow autistic patients to achieve what is possible within their abilities. Opportunities may be provided by paid jobs in sheltered work settings and 'on the job training' facilities. Projects have also been established that involve autistic people living with more or less intensive supervision by a professional and attending training centres to help them learn to live independently.

2.5 Drug Treatment

Drug treatment can play an important role in the treatment of distressing or maladaptive target symptoms such as hyperactivity, aggression, excitement, negativism, and ritualised, stereotyped or self-injurious behaviours. Furthermore, clinicians should not hesitate to treat comorbid disorders, such as major depressive disorder or bipolar disorder, with drugs. Drug treatment, however, should never be considered as the only intervention, and should always be part of a wider multidisciplinary treatment approach.

3. Drug Treatment Options

When starting medication, it is important to select appropriate targets of treatment and to monitor efficacy and adverse effects regularly. The biochemical basis for autism is not clear and clinicians began prescribing many drugs on the basis of pragmatic and empirical evidence. Parallel to clinical practice, ongoing research on neurotransmitter function in autism has provided new insight into drugs already in use and challenging hypotheses on newly introduced compounds.

3.1 Antipsychotics

3.1.1 Haloperidol

Haloperidol is the antipsychotic that has been most intensively studied in autism. In a series of controlled investigations the drug significantly decreased motor stereotypies, hyperactivity, withdrawal and negativism in a group of 2- to 8-year-old autistic children.[22,23] The dosage was individually obtained, and the optimal dosage (0.25 to 4.0 mg/day for 4 weeks) caused no discernible sedation. Two open studies[24,25] claim favourable results with haloperidol in children with PDD-NOS. The long term efficacy of haloperidol is not well documented,[26] although Perry et al.[27] found that after 6 months of treatment, haloperidol remained effective in 71.5% of children (20% remained unchanged and 8.5% worsened).

Adverse effects that have been reported with the use of haloperidol include dystonic reactions, acute dyskinesias, parkinsonism, akathisia, and autonomous and cardiovascular signs and symptoms. The advice in prescribing is 'start low, go slow'. Acute overdose in young autistic children does not always present with sedation, but more often with regression and disorganisation of behaviour, irritability and lowered frustration tolerance.[28] Although extrapyramidal symptoms (EPS) have been reported, antiparkinsonian medication should not be added on a routine basis. Tardive or withdrawal dyskinesias can also cause concern with long term haloperidol treatment. Of 82 autistic children treated with haloperidol for 6 months in a prospective study, 24 developed dyskinesias.[29] Tardive dyskinesias occurred in 5 patients, and withdrawal dyskinesias in 19. All the dyskinesia symptoms disappeared spontaneously or after discontinuation of haloperidol.

3.1.2 Other Antipsychotics

Despite the extensive body of data on the use of haloperidol in autism, most clinicians now use other antipsychotics as first-line treatments, given the frequency of severe adverse effects associated with haloperidol treatment. Pimozide proved to be as effective as haloperidol in a multicentre controlled trial.[30] It was also found to decrease hypoactivity in withdrawn in autistic children.[31] The therapeutic dosage ranges from 0.25 to 4 mg/day.

The role of atypical antipsychotics (which carry a lower risk of inducing EPS and have a stronger potential to affect the core social deficits of individuals with autism) has been investigated, although there have been no controlled studies with these agents as yet. Open label studies have documented promising clinical improvements following treatment with risperidone. For example, Hardan et al.[32] treated 20 children and adolescents who had a developmental disorder that was refractory to other psychotropic treatments with risperidone in dosages ranging from 1.5 to 10 mg/day. Risperidone decreased a wide range of symptoms, including psychosis, aggression, impulsivity, self-injurious behaviour and hyperactivity. Adverse effects reported were excessive bodyweight gain and galactorrhoea. McDougle et al.[33] treated 18 patients (mean age 10.2 ± 3.7 years) who had pervasive developmental disorders with risperidone. The optimal dosage was found to be 1.8 ± 1 mg/day. 12 of the patients were considered to be responders. A significant improvement was seen in measures of interfering repetitive behaviours, aggression and impulsivity, and some elements of impaired social relatedness. The most common adverse effect was bodyweight gain.

Risperidone has been associated with some cases of tardive dyskinesia: we recently dealt with 2 boys with autism who developed tardive dyskinesia while receiving risperidone. Both boys had symptoms in the oro-buccal region, which disappeared some weeks after risperidone was discontinued.

3.2 Selective Serotonin Reuptake Inhibitors

There is some rationale for treating patients who have autism with selective serotonin (5-hydroxytryptamine; 5-HT) reuptake inhibitors (SSRIs). At a descriptive level, the repetitive and ritualistic stereotyped behaviour patterns in autism are similar to the symptoms of patients with obsessive-compulsive disorder. 40 to 60% of patients with obsessive-compulsive disorder respond to treatment with SSRIs.[34] Furthermore, the only biochemical abnormality consistently associated with autism is hyperserotoninamia, which is found in 30 to 40% of all autistic patients.[35,36]

3.2.1 Clomipramine

Clomipramine is a tricyclic antidepressant and a potent nonselective serotonin reuptake inhibitor. Treatment with clomipramine in an open-label study[37] brought about promising improvements in social relatedness, obsessive-compulsive symptoms, and aggressive and impulsive behaviour in 4 of 5 autistic patients aged between 13 and 33 years. However, the therapeutic effects of clomipramine seem to be less clear in young children with autism.[21,38] Since treatment with clomipramine resulted in a high rate of adverse effects, such as a grand mal seizure (as a result of a reduction in seizure threshold), anticholinergic and cardiovascular adverse effects and behavioural toxicity, TCAs should be used judiciously in children with autism.

3.2.2 Fluvoxamine

Fluvoxamine proved significantly more effective than placebo in a recent 12-week, double-blind, placebo-controlled trial of 30 autistic adults.[39] Of the 15 patients who received fluvoxamine, 8 were categorised as responders. Other than mild sedation and nausea, fluvoxamine was well tolerated. However, a similar study with fluvoxamine in patients younger than 18 years of age could not establish a significant treatment response, and documented a high rate of adverse effects and adverse behavioural activation (J.C. McDougle, personal communication).

3.2.3 Fluoxetine

In a placebo-controlled study of 5 autistic patients aged between 10 and 30 years,[40] 1 participant showed a moderate improvement in compulsive symptoms when treated with fluoxetine 20 mg/day. In an open trial, 2 participants showed clinical improvement with fluoxetine 40 mg/day.[40] Treatment for longer than 18 months gave a sustained medication response in 2 of the 3 patients. However, none of the patients showed an improvement in the core symptoms of autism.

In summary, the results of SSRI treatment in adults with autism, who are characterised by strong behavioural rigidity and obsessive-compulsive–like symptoms, are encouraging. In contrast, children and adolescents seem to be very sensitive to the stimulating effects of SSRIs and have a much lower response rate.

3.3 Other Serotonergic Drugs

3.3.1 Fenfluramine

Initial studies with fenfluramine, a halogenated amphetamine that promotes the release and inhibits the reuptake of serotonin and blocks dopamine receptors, reported dramatic improvements in patients with autism.[41,42] This led to the initiation of a large multicentre trial and a number of independent controlled trials.[43] However, the results of these studies were mixed, and the initial claims could not be supported. This lack of efficacy, coupled with the potential neurotoxicity of fenfluramine[44] and the reports of serious adverse effects,[45] suggest that fenfluramine should not be recommended for clinical use.[46]

3.3.2 Buspirone

Buspirone has, to our knowledge, been used only in open studies in patients with autism. Buspirone is an agonist of the serotonin 5-HT$_{1A}$ receptor and has anxiolytic and mildly antidepressant properties. Realmuto et al.[47] treated 4 autistic children aged between 9 and 10 years with buspirone 5mg three times daily for 4 weeks. Two children showed clinical improvements, and no adverse effects were reported. When Ratey et al.[48] treated 14 developmentally disabled patients with buspirone 15 to 45 mg/day, 9 of them showed a decrease in anxiety, temper tantrums, aggression and self-injurious behaviour. We have successfully used buspirone (at dosages ranging from 15 to 30 mg/day) as an adjuvant in the residential treatment of disorganised and hyperaroused children with autism. Positive drug responses consisted of a reduction in affective lability and a decrease in primitive anxieties (such as a fear of the dark, thunder, etc.) and sleep disorders.

3.4 Opioid Receptor Antagonists

Panksepp[49] hypothesised that autism was caused by hyperfunction of the endogenous opioid system, resulting in diminished social interest. This prompted research into the therapeutic effects of opioid receptor antagonists in autism. However, 3 recent placebo-controlled studies in children with autism, using naltrexone, an orally active opioid antagonist, gave disappointing results.[50-53] Although treatment with naltrexone 1.0 mg/kg/day was consistently associated with a significant but modest reduction in hyperactivity, social and communicative deficits and stereotyped behaviours were not ameliorated. Also, open-label continuation treatment for 6 months with 5 of the children, who showed a clear individual response to naltrexone in the 4-week trial, did not show therapeutic effects on social and communicative functioning.[53] Furthermore, in a recent double-blind, placebo-controlled, crossover study in mentally retarded adults with autism and/or self-injurious behaviour, naltrexone failed to affect self-injurious and autistic behaviour in a positive way.[54] Adverse effects of naltrexone were mild and transient. Naltrexone has a bitter taste, which can give rise to compliance problems. On balance, we would not advocate routine use of naltrexone for the treatment of autism.

3.5 Stimulants

Psychostimulants are the first-line tools for the treatment of symptoms of hyperactivity, inattentiveness and impulsivity. Since patients with autism are often hyperactive and highly distractible, treatment with stimulants would appear an obvious strategy. Earlier studies found that methylphenidate worsened symptoms such as stereotypies when used in hyperactive children with autism.[55,56] A recent double-blind, placebo-controlled, crossover study of 10 children with autism aged between 7 and 11 years showed that methylphenidate 10 or 20mg twice daily resulted in a significant decrease in hyperactivity. Adverse effects, including worsening of stereotypic movements, were absent.[57] Adverse effects of stimulants are thought to occur mostly in mentally retarded children who have intelligence quotients below 45 or who have mental ages below 4.5 years.[58]

3.6 Clonidine

Two controlled studies[59,60] reported on the use of clonidine, an agonist of the presynaptic α_2-adrenergic receptor, in patients with autism. Short term use of clonidine reduced hyperactivity, impulsivity and irritability. However, clinical experience indicates that many patients develop tolerance to the therapeutic effects of clonidine, which limits the applicability of the drug in clinical practice. Reported adverse effects are an increase in drowsiness, decreased activity and hypotension.

Table I. Clinical guidelines for drug treatment in autism

Target	Agent	Studied in	Status
Inattentiveness, hyperactivity	Methylphenidate	Children	Clinical
	Antipsychotics	Children, adolescents	Clinical
	Clonidine	Children, adolescents, adults	Clinical
Rigidity, rituals	SSRIs	Children, adolescents, adults	Clinical
	Antipsychotics	Children, adolescents	Clinical
Aggression, self-injury	Antipsychotics	Children, adolescents	Clinical
	Lithium	Children, adolescents	Clinical
	β-Blockers	Adolescents, adults	Experimental
	Clonidine	Children, adolescents	Clinical
Anxiety, affective dysregulation	Buspirone	Children, adolescents	Clinical
	Antipsychotics	Children, adolescents	Clinical
	Clonidine	Children, adolescents	Clinical
Social impairments	Atypical antipsychotics	Children, adolescents, adults	Experimental

SSRIs = selective serotonin (5-hydroxytryptamine; 5-HT) reuptake inhibitors.

3.7 Propranolol

Propranolol, a lipophilic β-blocker, was used in open trials to treat aggression, self-injury and impulsivity in patients with developmental disorders.[61,62] The drug had favourable effects on aggressive and stereotypes behaviour, attention and communication. It is necessary to take an ECG recording before treatment starts and to monitor pulse rate and blood pressure regularly, because of the risk of bradycardia and hypotension.

3.8 Lithium

When the symptoms of autism show a cyclic pattern, or when a bipolar mood disorder is suspected, treatment with lithium can be helpful. Successful treatment with lithium of patients who have a periodic increase of autism symptoms has been described.[63,64] Lithium can also be used in the treatment of aggressive and self-injurious behaviour in patients with autism.[65]

3.9 Anticonvulsants

Twenty to 30% of children with an autistic disorder also experience symptoms of epilepsy. Therefore, anticonvulsants can play a role in the management of the disorder. As well as an anticonvulsant effect, carbamazepine is reported to have positive effects in mood disorders and on aggressive, irritative or explosive behaviour in autistic children.[66] Open label treatment with valproic acid (sodium valproate) also resulted in an improvement in behavioural symptoms associated with autism.[67]

4. Conclusion

Clinical guidelines for the drug treatment of autism are summarised in table I. When treating inattentiveness and hyperactivity, it is important to differentiate between: (i) a lack of social attention associated with joint attention deficits, one of the core impairments in autism; (ii) rigidity and preoccupation with particular interests; and (iii) distractibility in a task-related context similar to that observed in attention-deficit hyperactivity disorder. Only the latter type of problem is likely to benefit from treatment with methylphenidate. Alternative agents for treating inattentiveness and hyperactivity are antipsychotics and clonidine. Obsessive-compulsive–like symptoms and extreme behavioural rigidity in adults with autism may respond to SSRIs or antipsychotics; in children and adolescents with autism SSRIs should be used with great caution. Symptoms of self-injury and aggression may be treated with anti-psychotics, lithium, β-blocking agents or clonidine. Buspirone, antipsychotics or clonidine are options for treating patients experiencing primitive anxieties, affective dysregulation and sleep disturbances. When prescribing an antipsychotic, compounds such as pimozide or risperidone should generally be favoured over haloperidol, given the adverse effect profile of the latter. Last but not least, social relatedness and communicative impairments may be improved by the administration of atypical antipsychotics such as risperidone.

References

1. Kanner L. Autistic disturbances of affective contact. Nervous Child 1943; 2: 217-50
2. World Health Organization. The ICD-10 classification of mental and behavioural disorders: clinical descriptions and diagnostic guidelines. Geneva: World Health Organization, 1992
3. American Psychiatric Association. Diagnostic and statistical manual of mental disorders. 4th ed. Washington, DC: American Psychiatric Association, 1994
4. Bailey A, Philips W, Rutter M. Autism: towards an integration of clinical, genetic, neuropsychological, and neurobiological perspectives. J Child Psychol Psychiatry 1996; 37: 89-126
5. Wing L. The definition and prevalence of autism: a review. Eur Child Adolesc Psychiatry 1993; 2: 61-74
6. Lord C, Rutter M. Autism and pervasive developmental disorders. In: Rutter M, Taylor E, Hersov L, editors. Child and adolescent psychiatry: modern approaches. 3rd ed. Oxford: Blackwell Science Ltd, 1994: 569-93
7. Baron-Cohen S, Allen J, Gillberg C. Can autism be detected at 18 months? The needle, the haystack, and the CHAT. Br J Psychiatry 1992; 161: 839-43
8. Gillberg C, Nordin V, Ehlers S. Early detection of autism: diagnostic instruments for clinicians. Eur Child Adolesc Psychiatry 1996; 5: 67-74
9. Schopler E, Reichler RJ, Renner BR. The childhood autism rating scale (CARS) revised. Los Angeles: Western Psychological Services Inc., 1988
10. Lord C, Rutter M, Le Couteur A. Autism diagnostic interview-revised: a revised version of a diagnostic interview for caregivers of individuals with possible pervasive developmental disorders. J Autism Dev Discord 1994; 24: 659-85
11. Lord C, Rutter M, Goode S, et al. Autism diagnostic observation schedule: a standardized observation of communicative and social behavior. J Autism Dev Discord 1989; 19: 185-212
12. Gillberg C, Coleman M. Autism and medical disorders: a review of the literature. Dev Med Child Neurol 1996; 38: 191-202
13. Rutter M, Bailey A, Bolton P, et al. Autism and known medical conditions: myth and substance. J Child Psychol Psychiatry 1994; 35: 311-22
14. Rutter M. The treatment of autistic children. J Child Psychol Psychiatry 1985; 26 (2): 193-214
15. Van der Gaag RJ. Multiplex developmental disorder: an exploration of borderlines on the autistic spectrum [thesis]. Utrecht: University of Utrecht, 1993
16. Campbell M, Schopler E. Pervasive developmental disorders. In: Treatments of psychiatric disorders: a task force report of the American Psychiatric Association. Vol 1. Washington, DC: American Psychiatric Association, 1989: 201-17
17. Williams T. A social skills group for autistic children. J Autism Dev Discord 1989; 19: 143-56
18. Mesibov GB. Social skills training with verbal autistic adolescents and adults: a program model. J Autism Dev Discord 1984; 14: 395-404
19. Lovaas OI. Behavioral treatment and normal educational and intellectual functioning in young autistic children. J Consult Clin Psychol 1987; 55: 3-9
20. McEachin J, Smith T, Lovaas O. Long-term outcome for children with autism who received early intensive behavioral treatment. Am J Ment Retard 1993; 97: 359-72
21. Campbell M, Schopler E, Cueva JE, et al. Treatment of autistic disorder. J Am Acad Child Adolesc Psychiatry 1996; 35 (2): 134-43
22. Anderson LT, Campbell M, Graga DM, et al. Haloperidol in the treatment of infantile autism: effects on learning and behavioral symptoms. Am J Psychiatry 1984; 141: 1195-202
23. Anderson LT, Campbell M, Adams P, et al. The effects of haloperidol on discrimination learning and behavioral symptoms in autistic children. J Autism Dev Discord 1989; 19: 227-39
24. Fisher W, Kerbeshian J, Burd L. A treatable language disorder: pharmacological treatment of pervasive developmental disorder. J Dev Behav Pediatr 1986; 7: 73-6
25. Joshi PT, Capozzoli JA, Coyle JT. Low-dose neuroleptic therapy for children with childhood-onset pervasive developmental disorder. Am J Psychiatry 1988; 145: 335-8
26. Gilman JT, Tuchman RF. Autism and associated behavioral disorders: pharmacotherapeutic intervention. Ann Pharmacother 1995; 29: 47-56

27. Perry R, Campbell M, Adams P, et al. Long-term efficacy of haloperidol in autistic children: continuous versus discontinuous administration. J Am Acad Child Adolesc Psychiatry 1989; 28: 87-92
28. Campbell M, Anderson LT, Green WH, et al. Psychopharmacology. In: Cohen DJ, Donnellan AM, editors. Handbook of autism and pervasive developmental disorders. New York: Wiley & Sons, 1987: 545-65
29. Campbell M, Adams P, Perry R, et al. Tardive and withdrawal dyskinesia in autistic children: a prospective study. Psychopharmacol Bull 1988; 24: 251-5
30. Naruse H, Nagahata M, Nakane Y, et al. A multi-center double-blind trial of pimozide (Orap), haloperidol and placebo in children with behavioral disorders, using cross-over design. Acta Paedopsychiatr 1982; 48: 173-84
31. Ernst M, Magee HJ, Gonzalez NM, et al. Pimozide in autistic children. Psychopharmacol Bull 1992; 28: 187-91
32. Hardan A, Johnson K, Johnson C, et al. Case study: risperidone treatment of children and adolescents with developmental disorders. J Am Acad Child Adolesc Psychiatry 1996; 35 (11): 1551-6
33. McDougle CJ, Holmes JP, Bronson ME, et al. Risperidone treatment of children and adolescents with pervasive developmental disorders: a prospective open-label study. J Am Acad Child Adolesc Psychiatry 1997; 36: 685-93
34. Greist JH, Jefferson JW, Kobak KA, et al. Efficacy and tolerability of serotonin transport inhibitors in obsessive-compulsive disorder. Arch Gen Psychiatry 1995; 52: 53-60
35. Anderson GM, Horne WC, Chatterjee D, et al. The hyperserotonemia of autism. Ann NY Acad Sci 1990; 600: 331-42
36. Cook EHJ, Leventhal BL, Heller W, et al. Autistic children and their first-degree relatives: relationships between serotonin and norepinephrine levels and intelligence. J Neuropsychiatry Clin Neurosci 1990; 2: 268-74
37. McDougle CJ, Price LH, Volkmar FR, et al. Clomipramine in autism: preliminary evidence of efficacy (case study). J Am Acad Child Adolesc Psychiatry 1992; 31: 746-50
38. Sanchez LE, Campbell M, Small AM, et al. A pilot study of clomipramine in young autistic children. J Am Acad Child Adolesc Psychiatry 1996; 35 (4): 537-44
39. McDougle CJ, Naylor ST, Cohen DJ, et al. A double blind, placebo-controlled study of fluvoxamine in adults with autistic disorder. Arch Gen Psychiatry 1996; 53: 1001-8
40. Bregman J, Volkmar F, Cohen DJ. Fluoxetine in the treatment of autistic disorder [abstract]. Proceedings of the 38th Annual Meeting of the American Academy of Child and Adolescent Psychiatry; 1991, 52
41. Geller E, Ritvo ER, Freeman BJ. Preliminary observations on the effects of fenfluramine on blood serotonin and symptoms in three autistic boys. N Engl J Med 1982; 307: 165-9
42. Ritvo ER, Freeman BJ, Geller E, et al. Effects of fenfluramine on 14 outpatients with the syndrome of autism. J Am Acad Child Psychiatry 1983; 22: 549-58
43. Ritvo ER, Freeman BJ, Yuwiler A, et al. Fenfluramine treatment of autism: UCLA collaboration study of 81 patients at nine medical centers. Psychopharmacol Bull 1986; 22: 133-40
44. Schuster CR, Lewis M, Seiden LS. Fenfluramine: neurotoxicity. Psychopharmacol Bull 1986; 22: 148-51
45. Realmuto GM, Jensen J, Klykylo W, et al. Untoward effects of fenfluramine in autistic children. J Clin Psychopharmacol 1986; 6: 350-5
46. Buitelaar JK. Psychopharmacological approaches to childhood psychotic disorders. In: Den Boer JA, Westenberg HGM, van Praag HM, editors. Advances in the neurobiology of schizophrenia. New York: Wiley & Sons, 1995: 429-57
47. Realmuto GM, August GJ, Garfinkel BD. Clinical effect of buspirone in autistic children. J Clin Psychopharmacol 1989; 9: 122-5
48. Ratey JJ, Sovner R, Mikkelsen E, et al. Buspirone therapy for maladaptive behavior and anxiety in developmentally disabled persons. J Clin Psychiatry 1989; 50: 382-4
49. Panksepp J. A neurochemical theory of autism. Trends Neurosci 1979; 2: 174-7
50. Campbell M, Anderson LT, Small AM, et al. Naltrexone in autistic children: behavioral symptoms and attentional learning. J Am Acad Child Adolesc Psychiatry 1993; 32: 1283-91
51. Kolmen BK, Feldman HM, Handen BL, et al. Naltrexone in young autistic children: a double-blind, placebo-controlled crossover study. J Am Acad Child Adolesc Psychiatry 1995; 34: 223-31
52. Willemsen-Swinkels SHN, Buitelaar JK, Weijnen FG, et al. Placebo-controlled acute dosage naltrexone study in young autistic children. Psychiatry Res 1995; 58: 203-15
53. Willemsen-Swinkels SHN, Buitelaar JK, Van Engeland H. The effects of chronic naltrexone treatment in young autistic children: a double-blind placebo-controlled crossover study. Biol Psychiatry 1996; 39: 1023-31
54. Willemsen-Swinkels SHN, Buitelaar JK, Nijhof G, et al. Failure of naltrexone to reduce autistic and self-injurious behavior in mentally retarded adults. Arch Gen Psychiatry 1995; 52: 766-73
55. Campbell M, Fish B, David R, et al. Response to triiodothyronine and dextroamphetamine: a study of preschool schizophrenic children. J Autism Child Schizophr 1972; 2: 343-57
56. Bloom AS, Russel LJ, Weisskopf B, et al. Methylphenidate- induced delusional disorder in a child with attention-deficit disorder with hyperactivity (case study). J Am Acad Child Adolesc Psychiatry 1988; 27: 88-9
57. Quintana H, Birmaher B, Stedge D, et al. Use of methylphenidate in the treatment of children with autistic disorder. J Autism Dev Discord 1995; 25 (3): 283-94
58. Aman MG, Marks RE, Turbott SH, et al. Clinical effects of methylphenidate and thioridazine in intellectually sub-average children. J Am Acad Child Adolesc Psychiatry 1991; 30: 246-56
59. Fankhauser MP, Karumanchi VC, German ML, et al. A double-blind, placebo-controlled study of the efficacy of transdermal clonidine in autism. J Clin Psychiatry 1992; 53: 77-82
60. Jaselskis C, Cook EH, Fletcher KE, et al. Clonidine treatment of hyperactive and impulsive children with autistic disorder. J Clin Psychopharmacol 1992; 12: 322-7

61. Ratey JJ, Bemporad J, Sorgi P, et al. Brief report: open trial effects of beta-blockers on speech and social behaviors in 8 autistic adults. J Autism Dev Discord 1987; 17: 439-46
62. Ratey JJ, Mikkelsen E, Sorgi P, et al. Autism: the treatment of aggressive behaviors. J Clin Psychopharmacol 1987; 7: 35-41
63. Komoto JM, Usui S, Hirata J. Infantile autism and affective disorder. J Autism Dev Discord 1984; 14: 81-4
64. Kerbeshian J, Burd L, Fisher W. Lithium carbonate in the treatment of two patients with infantile autism and atypical bipolar symptomatology. J Clin Psychopharmacol 1987; 7: 401-5
65. Buitelaar JK. Self-injurious behavior in retarded children, clinical phenomena and biological mechanisms. Acta Paedopsychiatr 1993; 56: 105-12
66. Gillberg C. The treatment of epilepsy in autism. J Autism Dev Discord 1991; 21: 61-77
67. Plioplys A. Autism: electroencephalographic abnormalities and clinical improvement with valproic acid. Arch Pediatr Adolesc Med 1994; 148: 220-2

Correspondence: Prof. *Jan K. Buitelaar*, Department of Child Psychiatry, P.O. Box 85500, 3508 GA Utrecht, The Netherlands.
E-mail: J.K.Buitelaar@psych.azu.nl

Learning Disabilities
Classification, Clinical Features and Treatment

Yitzchak Frank

Division of Pediatric Neurology, Departments of Neurology and Pediatrics,
North Shore University Hospital, Cornell University Medical College, Manhasset,
New York, USA

1. History and Definition

Learning disabilities are manifested by a variety of academic problems, including reading disability (dyslexia), and problems with mathematics and written expression.[1-6] Deficits of organisational skills and motor performance, although not traditionally listed among academic difficulties, are also common. Although the most common form of disability is that of reading, many patients with learning disabilities have a mixture of academic problems.

Descriptions of learning disabilities date back at least 100 years.[7-8] The name of this condition and its definition have changed a number of times. The names 'minimal brain damage' and 'minimal brain dysfunction' reflect the hypothesis that the condition is neuro- logical in origin. These terms are also derived from the observation that children affected by the influenza encephalitis epidemic of 1918 in the US manifested, among other neurological abnormalities, hyperactivity, short attention span and learning difficulties.[9]

A definition by a US National Advisory Committee on Handicapped Children in 1968, used in Public Law 94-142 (the law mandating education to all handicapped children), made an important step in the direction of endorsing a biological basis for learning disabilities. This definition relates learning disabilities to a disorder of basic psychological processes involved in the understanding or in the use of language.[10]

The current definition of learning disorders in DSM-IV reads: 'Learning disorders are diagnosed when the individual's achievement on individually administered, standardised tests in reading, mathematics, or written expression is substantially below that expected for age, schooling, and level of intelligence'.[11] It differentiates this group of disorders from learning disorders resulting from impaired vision or hearing, social or emotional disturbance, cultural differences, or insufficient or inappropriate instruction. Learning disability does not refer to an inability to learn resulting from mental retardation or communication disorders.

Underlying abnormalities of one or more selected cognitive processes are frequently present in individuals with learning disability, including language processing, visual perception or memory abnormalities, and are presumably responsible for the learning difficulties. Other cognitive abilities may be normal, or even superior, in the same children. Although these cognitive abnormalities underlying learning disabilities are frequently present from birth, the disorder is usually detected at the onset of formal education in school.

Children with learning disabilities differ in the degree of their difficulties, in general intelligence and in comorbid conditions, all of which are important both for treatment and prognosis.

2. Prevalence

Learning disability is one of the most common neurobehavioural disorders. Estimates of the prevalence of learning disabilities vary, but are conservatively in the range of 3 to 6% of the childhood population.[12] When attention deficit hyperactivity disorder (ADHD) is included among the learning disabilities, the prevalence at least doubles. The Isle of Wight study estimated that 4% of the study population had a specific reading disability.[13,14] A study by Shaywitz et al.[15] found that the prevalence of reading disability among Connecticut school children was 6 to 9%.

Some studies have shown that learning disabilities and reading disability are much more prevalent in boys than in girls, with boys : girls ratios of 2 : 1 to 5 : 1.[1,16] However, the Connecticut study[15] found no significant difference in prevalence between males and females. The authors suggested that school-identified samples are biased towards a higher prevalence of boys.

A specific mathematical disability is, by itself, much less common, with a prevalence of about 1%, and the majority of mathematically disabled children may have other deficits (i.e. in social skills).[17]

3. Classification

Learning disabilities are classified in DSM-IV according to the type of academic difficulty (i.e. reading disability, mathematical disability, expressive writing disability). Although such a classification seems practical to educators, it may be misleading because learning disability syndromes may frequently include mixed symptomatology.

A more precise classification is a clinical-neuropsychological one,[2] which recognises five types of learning disorder based on abnormalities of: (i) phonological processing; (ii) spatial cognition; (iii) executive functions; (iv) social recognition; and (v) long term memory. It is suggested that each type of learning disability represents a localised developmental abnormality of a brain system: left perisylvia, right hemisphere, frontal lobes, limbic system and right hemisphere, and hippocampus and amygdala, respectively. However, the biological validation of these syndromes has only recently been undertaken.

The abnormality of phonological processing-type learning disability is probably a developmental language disorder, and will cause reading disability.[18]

Spatial cognition abnormality-type learning disability is manifested by problems of visual and spatial memory, recognition and construction, and object localisation and identification,[19] causing the 'right hemisphere learning disability' syndrome. These children have greater problems with mathematics and psychosocial adjustment than with reading and spelling. This type of learning disability is much less prevalent than that of the phonological processing-type, constituting about 10% of a learning disabilities clinic population.[20] However, it is also probably underdiagnosed.

The executive functions abnormality-type learning disability is manifested by difficulties with planning, organisational skills, selective attention and inhibitory control. The prefrontal brain areas appear to be specialised for these functions.[21,22] This syndrome is also known as

ADHD. Affected children may have hyperactivity, a short attention span, high distractibility and impulsivity affecting their academic achievements and social contacts.

The social cognition abnormality-type learning disability needs more validation, as well as distinction from other syndromes characterised by social and communication abnormalities including Asperger's syndrome, pervasive developmental disorders and the right hemisphere learning disability syndrome.

Similarly, it is not clear that the long term memory-type learning disability, which is hypothetically the result of developmental abnormalities involving the hippocampus, amygdala, basal ganglia and the cerebellum, has independent symptomatology.

4. Aetiology

Initial descriptions of 'word blindness' assumed that developmental reading disability is caused by focal brain damage, similar to the model of alexia in adults. However, learning disabilities can result from a number of conditions affecting the CNS in early life.

Hypoxic-ischemic encephalopathy, infection or trauma can cause learning disabilities. In most such cases, there will be an appropriate history as well as other neurological abnormalities, including motor abnormalities. Learning disabilities are common in children with neurofibromatosis,[23] early-treated phenylketonuria,[24] abnormally high lead levels,[25,26] and seizures.

A selective language-based reading disability is prevalent among children with a 47 XXY karyotype.[27]

An association between left-handedness, reading disability, immune disorders and migraine has been proposed.[28] It has been suggested that testosterone *in utero* leads to abnormal development of left hemisphere dominance, resulting in left-handedness and developmental language disorders and learning disabilities, and to anomalous development of the immune system leading to autoimmune and atopic illnesses later in life.[28,29]

However, at least one-third of the cases of learning disabilities are probably familial.[30] Reports of learning disabilities or reading abnormalities in more than one family member appeared as early as 1905, and have led to the suggestion of a genetic transmission of reading difficulty.[31-34] Transmission may be variable and the disorder is genetically heterogeneous.[35] It is possible that the inherited trait is a more basic neuropsychological abnormality that is an important component of reading acquisition. An example of such an inherited trait is phonological coding, a measure of the knowledge of the sound structure of the language. This is more likely to be abnormal in monozygotic than in dizygotic twin pairs with reading disability.[36]

An abnormality of the short limb of chromosome 15 in some families with reading disability was reported in 1983.[37] However, further research has shown evidence for a linkage on chromosome 6 in the human leucocyte antigen region.[38]

5. Comorbidity

A definite comorbidity exists between learning disabilities and ADHD, a neurobehavioural syndrome characterised by developmentally inappropriate degrees of inattention, impulsivity and overactivity. More than one-half of children with ADHD have learning disabilities.[39-41] Some authors classify ADHD as a type of learning disability, the executive functions abnormality-type (see section 3).[2]

Children with learning disabilities may also have a comorbid conduct disorder, symptoms of depression (dysthymia), or other behavioural and emotional disturbances. Children with nonverbal learning disabilities frequently have social skills abnormalities as a part of their disorder.[42]

6. Biological Correlates

6.1 Anatomy

In an unselected autopsy population, the planum temporale (a region of the posterior superior surface of the temporal lobe auditory cortex involved with auditory comprehension) was usually asymmetrical, being larger on the left in 65% of cases, larger on the right in 10% of cases and symmetrical in only 25% of cases.[43] Planum asymmetry has been documented as early as 33 weeks of gestation.[44,45] In contrast, a lack of such asymmetry was found in the brains of patients with learning disabilities. In addition, multiple foci of cerebral microdysgenesis or ectopias, including focal microgyria and nests of neurons and gliosis, were found in the brains of reading-disabled patients, while the brains of unaffected controls showed only few such changes.[46]

It was suggested that loss of planum temporale asymmetry is caused by increased numbers of neurons in the right side, while microdysgenesis results from prenatal injury during the migration stage of brain development. The nature of the presumed prenatal injury is not clear. However, it has been proposed, based on animal research, that autoimmune damage of vessel walls caused reduced blood flow, mainly in 'watershed' parts of the developing cortex, leading to the cortical injury, scars and malformations.[47,48]

Computerised tomography (CT) brain scans demonstrated a reversal of the usual brain asymmetry in some patients, but in general failed to show consistent abnormalities.[49] Magnetic resonance imaging (MRI) studies revealed a lack of planum temporale asymmetry, but also exaggerated asymmetries in the temporal and parietal lobes.[50-52]

A positron emission tomography (PET) study of regional metabolic activity during oral reading in right-handed men with and without a childhood family history of reading disability, demonstrated a different pattern of brain activation in patients with reading disability. In contrast to the asymmetry observed in the prefrontal and the lingual regions in unaffected individuals during reading, the pattern was more symmetrical.[53]

Another study of brain metabolism in adults who were diagnosed with reading disability in childhood was performed during an auditory speech discrimination task. This revealed a different pattern of abnormal activation, with an unusually high metabolic rate in the medial temporal region, an area that contains afferent fibres believed to relay auditory stimulation to primary auditory processing centres. These results demonstrate that individuals who had familial developmental reading disability as children, activate different brain regions during reading as adults compared with individuals without such a childhood history.[54] Similarly, Shaywitz et al.,[54a] using functional MRI, found that individuals with dyslexia have abnormal brain activation during reading with reduced activation of the left perisylvian and occipital areas and overactivation of the inferior frontal gyrus and right posterior perisylvian region.

6.2 Electrophysiology

The EEG may show nonspecific abnormalities in children with learning disabilities, including background disorganisation and slowing, and, infrequently, epileptiform abnormalities.

Studies of event-related potentials, which record averaged brain potentials elicited in response to stimuli, seemed very suitable to demonstrate perceptual abnormalities causing reading disability or learning disabilities. Early studies with brain electrical activity mapping – a topographical mapping of EEG and event-related potentials – identified differences between children with and without reading disabilities in both hemispheres, but maximally in left posterior areas and in both frontal areas.[55]

Other event-related potential studies demonstrated that individuals with reading disabilities activated the right hemisphere, instead of left hemisphere, in response to linguistic stimuli.[56] This finding supports a hypothesis that a relatively weak left hemisphere activation can underlie learning disabilities.[57]

Other studies show reduced amplitude of the P3 cognitive potential in children with learning disabilities.[58] Livingstone et al.,[59] using a different event-related potentials technique, found abnormalities (slower response) in a group of children with reading disabilities when fast, low contrast stimuli were presented. This type of stimuli is handled by the magnocellular pathway of the visual system. The magnocellular pathway starts at the retina and continues through to the lateral geniculate nucleus, the primary visual cortex and higher order visual cortices, and mediates the processing of rapid visual transitions at low contrasts. The other visual pathway – the parvocellular – which is slow, relatively contrast insensitive and colour selective, appeared to function normally in these children.

Timing of the evoked potentials abnormality found in the children with reading disabilities suggests that the abnormality is in the retina or the lateral geniculate nucleus. Measurement of neurons of the magno- and parvocellular layers of the lateral geniculate nucleus in 5 brains from individuals with reading disabilities and 5 control brains revealed smaller magno cells in those with reading disability, complementing the physiological findings of a slowed magnocellular system.[59]

The authors proposed that individuals with reading disability have a deficiency involving the fast processing of visual and auditory stimuli, interfering with efficient language processing when fast processing is required for extraction of meaning. Unfortunately, this study only involved a small number of patients and, as yet, has not been replicated.

In summary, the most consistently found biological abnormality has been anatomic – the lack of the normal left-larger-than-right asymmetry of the planum temporale section of the temporal lobe. The symmetry found in individuals with reading disability may represent relatively excessive numbers of neurons and interhemispheric connections in the right hemisphere[60,61] or a smaller left hemisphere.

Neurophysiological research has demonstrated an abnormal neuronal activation pattern in learning disabilities, but has not yet identified a persistent pattern. Studies of brain metabolism have also pointed to an unusual activation pattern during reading, but these need to be replicated. It is possible that improved study techniques and the selection of patients according to learning disability subtypes will elicit more specific and consistent biological abnormalities.

7. Evaluation

The symptoms leading to the referral of patients with learning disabilities for an evaluation vary according to the type of learning disability and the presence of comorbidities, and are also age-dependent. Academic underperformance is a common symptom leading to investigation, but comorbid disruptive behaviour symptomatology or inattention may be the predominant features. Adolescents may be referred because they avoid school or because they present with symptoms of depression.

7.1 History

A detailed school history, starting from nursery school, should be obtained. This should include time of onset, type and severity of difficulties, amount of time the child spends doing homework, and any academic help received at school or at home. Symptoms of attentional difficulties, inability to complete tasks, distractibility, hyperactivity and impulsiveness are important because of the frequent comorbidity of learning disabilities and ADHD. Any history of discipline problems, school avoidance, conduct disorder, oppositional defiant disorder, dysthymia and depression should be documented. Special behavioural forms completed by parents (i.e. the Conner's Parent Questionnaire and Achenbach Child behavioural Checklist) and teachers (Conner's Teacher's Questionnaire and Achenbach Teacher's Response Form) prior to the office visit can be of significant help in evaluating comorbid behavioural difficulties.

Social problems and low self-esteem are common in children with learning disabilities and should be documented. A general paediatric history should include a detailed developmental history, noting any encephalopathic event, speech and language abnormalities, and gross or fine motor milestones delay.[62] A history of speech delay or an inability to learn nursery rhymes is frequently present in reading-disabled children. A detailed family history including history of learning disabilities, pervasive developmental disorder, mental retardation or ADHD is important because of the frequent genetic origin of learning disabilities.

7.2 Physical Examination and Laboratory Tests

The general physical examination should note craniofacial malformations and asymmetries, increased head size, café au lait or depigmented skin areas, liver or spleen enlargement and retinal lesions, which may be associated with brain abnormalities giving rise to learning difficulties. Frequently observed neurological abnormalities in children with learning disabilities and ADHD are motor incoordination, pseudochoreoathetosis, mirror movements and disdiadochokinesis ('soft signs'). Timed motor coordination batteries can assist in detecting such abnormalities.[63]

There are no laboratory tests necessary for learning disabilities diagnosis. Radiological tests (i.e. MRI of the brain) and EEG may show an abnormality, but, as noted in section 6.2, lack the consistency and specificity needed for the individual diagnosis. These tests are done in some patients when a structural brain abnormality or a seizure disorder are suspected.

Similarly, blood and urine tests should be taken when a systemic abnormality is suspected. Our neurobehavioural clinic suggests a total blood count, a chemistry profile, thyroid functions and blood lead level assessment in all patients with a diagnosis of learning disabilities or ADHD.

Genetic consultation, including fragile X DNA testing and chromosomal analysis, should be done if dysmorphic features are present.

7.3 Academic Achievement Testing

The DSM-IV criteria for learning disorders provide the basis for diagnosis. The most common method for determining the existence of learning disabilities is to demonstrate a substantial discrepancy (1.5 to 2 standard deviations below the mean) between educational achievement and intellectual potential in one or more areas of learning. Another method assesses the number of years or months a child's academic performance lags behind grade level. Both methods entail the administration of standardised tests to measure both IQ and educational achievement.

A screen for learning disability can be done in the office and should include reading of an age-appropriate text, writing, spelling, a memory test and copying geometric shapes. However, the diagnosis of learning disabilities cannot be made without formal academic achievement (and neuropsychological) testing.

7.4 Neuropsychological Testing

Neuropsychological testing will usually be done by psychologists or neuro-psychologists and include measures of intelligence [i.e. Wechsler Intelligence Scale for Children (WISC-III) and the Stanford Binet Intelligence Scale, fourth edition], academic achievements in reading, writing, spelling and arithmetic [i.e. Kaufman Test of Educational Achievement-Comprehensive Form (K-TEA), Peabody Individual Achievement Test-Revised (PIAT-R), Woodcock-Johnson Tests of Achievement-Revised (WJ-R), and the Wide Range Achievement Test-Revised (WRAT-R)], and diverse cognitive testing. Cognitive and achievement tests should be chosen according to the patient's primary language, ethnic origin and cultural background.

Academic achievement tests will determine the presence of learning disabilities, while neuropsychological testing will frequently reveal the underlying cognitive abnormalities. Neuropsychological testing should include specific tests for language, memory, construction, visual motor coordination and 'executive functions', including attention, learning strategies and motor tests.[1]

Neuropsychological abnormalities described in learning disabilities are not uniform.[64] Those frequently found in reading disability are speech, language or verbal learning impairment. These range from global language dysfunction to more selective anomic, articulatory, dysphonemic or verbal memory deficits,[65] although particular language skills, like phonemic segmentation, may be more closely associated with reading.[66]

Abnormalities in visual naming speed in patients with reading disability have been described. In a study of a reading-disabled group of children, 90% could be neuropsychologically classified. Approximately 75% had speech and/or language disorders (i.e. articulatory and/or naming) and less than 25% had visual perceptual deficits. Graphomotor, articulatory and temporal sequencing abnormalities were also present.[67]

Emotional, behavioural and social adjustment should be evaluated to exclude a primary psychiatric disorder and to identify frequent comorbidities such as ADHD or depression.[68,69]

8. Treatment

The goals of treatment of children with learning disabilities are the achievement of academic competence, prevention of emotional problems and treatment of comorbid conditions (i.e. ADHD). Treatment modalities include academic help, psychotherapy and medications.

8.1 Educational-Cognitive Treatment

The primary treatment for learning disabilities is special education.[1,64] This should be school based, include slower and repetitive teaching, individually or in small groups, administered by special education teachers using appropriate techniques and teaching aids.[69-71] Educational modifications include allowance for more time to complete tests and assignments.[72]

The cognitive examination is instrumental in identifying the specific cognitive profile and disability of an individual child. The best approach to special education is to prepare an individual educational plan according to the student's neuropsychological deficits and skills. Reading-disabled children with language abnormalities may benefit from visual-type teaching. Traditional education may need to be supplemented with functional curricula, computers, vocational training or work study. Tutoring out of school is usually effective only in less severe cases.

The intensity of special education and the extent of 'mainstreaming' of the individual child with learning disabilities depends on the degree of the disability. In the most difficult cases a special class placement may be needed. The efficacy of specific remedial reading programmes for reading disability (i.e. the Orton-Gillingham, Distar or Stevenson reading programmes) has been debated. Few published reports provide any convincing evidence of significant treatment effects obtained with these methods. Teaching of phonological skills may be beneficial.

It is important to explain the diagnosis of learning disabilities and the individual difficulties to the student, family and teachers. The understanding that learning disabilities is an inherent disability and that the child is not 'stupid' or 'lazy' enhances self-esteem and usually improves behaviour and motivation.

8.2 Psychological Treatment

Psychological consequences of learning disorders stem from constant classroom failure, frequently accompanied by social difficulties, and include reduced self-esteem, anxiety and depressive features, which continue, in varied forms, into adult life.[73] The ongoing academic failure reduces the child's motivation to learn and some of them may refuse to go to school.

Reduced self-esteem may lead to provocative behaviours in the classroom, and to anger projected to teachers and parents. Efforts to build self-esteem may include special jobs within the classroom, sports, scouts, music, drama, arts and crafts, and other nonacademic activities where the child with learning disabilities may excel and will not differ from his or her peers.

Therapy may be in the form of individual, group or family therapy.[1] behavioural management techniques and social skills training are also used. Therapy sessions should be highly structured because many of the children are anxious or have ADHD. The therapist should also consider the child's cognitive difficulties, which frequently involve language problems.

8.3 Pharmacological Treatment

There is no known pharmacological treatment for learning disabilities. However, cholinergic agents, nootropic medications, ergoloid mesylates, central stimulants, catecholamines, opioids and pituitary-adrenal hormones may have an effect on memory and learning.[74] Some of these agents have been tried in patients with learning disabilities and conditions involving cognitive degeneration.[75]

8.3.1 Nootropics

Piracetam and oxiracetam are nootropic compounds that are structurally related to the neurotransmitter γ-aminobutyric acid (GABA).

While oxiracetam has not been assessed in patients with learning disabilities, it has been shown to have effects in patients with primary degenerative dementia. In such patients, treatment with oxiracetam 1600 mg/day resulted in an improvement of simple reaction time and cognitive functions measured by attention tests.[76] Oxiracetam was also found to improve the latency and amplitude of the P300 wave in cognitive-evoked potential studies.[77]

A multisite, 12-week, double-blind, placebo-controlled study of piracetam in boys with learning disabilities showed improved reading speed, but no significant effects on either reading accuracy or reading comprehension measures.[78] A longer (36 weeks) multisite evaluation reported small, but reliable, improvements in oral passage reading (accuracy and speed scores combined) for piracetam-treated children, but no improvement on the reading speed measure.[79] Most other measures of information processing, language and memory were not significantly improved with piracetam treatment. Another more recent study using piracetam in two subgroups of students with reading disability, 'dysphonetic' or 'phonetic', did not find an improvement in any aspect of reading.[80]

Table I provides the suggested dosage of piracetam for use in patients with learning disabilities.

Table I. Drugs that may be used in patients with learning disabilities

Drug	Dosage (mg/day)	Adverse effects	Target symptoms
Nootropic			
Piracetam	1000-3000	Mild dizziness, insomnia, nausea	Possible effects on reading skills
Central stimulants			
Methylphenidate	2.5-60	Decreased appetite, insomnia, stomach ache, headache, tics, growth suppression (long term use)	Symptoms of ADHD, possible indirect effects on learning
Dexamphetamine	2.5-40	Decreased appetite, insomnia, stomach ache, headache, tics, growth suppression (long term use)	Symptoms of ADHD, possible indirect effects on learning
Pemoline	37.5-75	Decreased appetite, insomnia, stomach ache, headache, tics, growth suppression (long term use), increased levels of liver enzymes	Symptoms of ADHD, possible indirect effects on learning
Clonidine	0.05-0.2	Sedation, hypotension, bradycardia, cardiac arrythmia, dermatitis (with transdermal system)	Hyperactivity, hyperarousal, tics
Antidepressants			
Desipramine	25-100	Drowsiness, anticholinergic and cardiovascular effects, bodyweight gain, irritability, gastrointestinal upset	Behavioural abnormalities, particularly features of depression or anxiety
Imipramine	20-100	Drowsiness, anticholinergic and cardiovascular effects, bodyweight gain, irritability, gastrointestinal upset	Behavioural abnormalities, particularly features of depression or anxiety
SSRIs	Fluoxetine 5-20	Gastrointestinal effects, sleep disturbances, nervousness, headache	Behavioural abnormalities, particularly features of depression or anxiety

116

8.3.2 Central Stimulants

In children with ADHD, stimulant medications improve classroom behaviour and learning, impulsivity, attention and social interaction, and the performance on cognitive laboratory tasks, such as continuous performance tasks testing vigilance, impulsivity and attention.[81,82] Comprehensive reviews of the use of stimulant medications in ADHD are available.[83-85]

When ADHD is a comorbid condition with learning disabilities, the main avenue of treatment is the stimulants, such as methylphenidate, dexamphetamine and pemoline (table I). The specific therapeutic mode of action of the stimulants is not clear, although they appear to increase release and decrease reuptake of neurotransmitters in central dopaminergic and noradrenergic systems.

Sustained-release tablets of methylphenidate and dexamphetamine are available and enable children to take single daily doses of medication (in the morning), avoiding the need for taking medication at school.[86] Some children will take a combination of both the sustained-release and immediate-release tablets.

Stimulants may improve classroom performance and therefore have an indirectly beneficial effect on learning. Classroom arithmetic tests were improved in individuals receiving methylphenidate.[87] It is not known, however, whether stimulants have a direct effect on learning or on long term academic achievements in children with learning disabilities.

It has been shown that with an increased dose of methylphenidate, behaviour and attention span may improve, but that the learning effect has a ceiling and actually may deteriorate.[88] A possible direct effect of stimulants on learning may therefore be masked by the dose given for behavioural control.

Pemoline is a long-acting stimulant, but a therapeutic effect may take 3 to 6 weeks to appear and 2% of children taking it may have abnormalities in liver function tests.[89]

Clonidine, an α-adrenergic receptor blocker, may be more effective in reducing hyperactivity and hyperarousal, while the stimulants have a more direct effect on distractibility and attention. Clonidine can be used as the medication of first-choice when tics are present. However, it may have a delayed onset of therapeutic effect, may have to be given 3 to 4 times per day and has important adverse effects (see table I).[90]

8.3.3. Antidepressants

Antidepressants can be used when other behavioural abnormalities, particularly features of depression or anxiety, are present (table I).[91-94]

Patients treated with these medications should be appropriately monitored, including blood pressure and pulse, blood cell count, liver and kidney functions and cardiac function. Blood concentrations for the tricyclic antidepressants are monitored to assure compliance and that concentrations remain within the therapeutic range.

Selective serotonin (5-hydroxytryptamine; 5-HT) reuptake inhibitors may have a similar therapeutic effect, although information on their use in children with learning disabilities, or learning disabilities and comorbid ADHD is still scarce.

9. Prognosis

Learning disability is a chronic condition that may continue into adolescence or adulthood, although the symptomatology may change. Learning abilities may improve over time with the acquisition of compensatory learning strategies, which may circumvent the specific difficulties. On the other hand, academic demands increase over time and there is an increased need for the organisational and study skills that children with learning disabilities frequently lack.[1]

It has been shown that children diagnosed with a reading disability at the beginning of primary school will still be below the standard level in reading at the end of this schooling period.[95-97] In some individuals, reading and spelling difficulties will continue into adulthood, although they may have good reading comprehension. In addition, several studies suggest that children with learning disabilities do less well as adults in areas of work and social and psychological adjustment.[98]

Emotional factors may be crucial in determining prognosis. Children with learning disabilities tend to develop emotional problems including a low self-esteem, oppositional tendencies and depressive symptoms.[99-101] As noted by Critchly,[7] 'The dyslexic is apt to find himself an alien in a critical, if not hostile, milieu; mocked, misunderstood, or penalised, cut off from opportunities for advancement'. The psychological reactions to this include clowning, aggressiveness and later delinquency. As a result, adolescents with learning disabilities are over-represented in the juvenile delinquency populations.[102]

The ultimate prognosis depends on the severity of the disability, the child's intelligence, the presence of ADHD and emotional abnormalities, the will and ability of the child to cope with the disability, and the environmental support of family and school. The prognosis of a learning-disabled child who can adapt him/herself to his/her disability and has no ADHD or other significant behavioural problem can be excellent, and although they may complete less formal education, they may be as successful as other adults.[1]

10. Conclusions

Learning disabilities are a common cause of academic, social and emotional problems in the school-aged child, and may hinder success in later life. These disabilities seem to be biologically and, frequently, genetically determined. However, there are no reliable biological tests, and the diagnosis is made primarily by measuring academic achievements and cognitive functions.

The first-line treatments for learning disabilities are educational-cognitive and psychological treatments; however, drug treatments also have a role in therapy. While there are no specific drugs that remedy learning disabilities, pharmacological therapy is aimed at improving comorbid conditions such as ADHD. Psychostimulants (i.e. methylphenidate or dexamphetamine) improve classroom behaviour and indirectly have a beneficial effect on learning. Antidepressants (i.e. imipramine and desipramine) improve other behavioural abnormalities, in particular depression and anxiety, which interfere with normal academic learning.

A better understanding of the specific types of learning disabilities and their underlying cognitive abnormalities, and the development of drugs that enhance learning and retention of learned material, will improve the chance for the successful treatment of learning disabilities.

References
1. Shapiro BK, Gallico RP. Learning disabilities. Pediatr Clin North Am 1993; 40: 490-505
2. Penington BF. Diagnosing learning disorders. A neuropsychological framework. New York: The Guilford Press, 1991
3. Shaywitz BA, Shaywitz SE. Learning disabilities and attention disorders. In: Swaiman KF, editor. Pediatric neurology, principles and practice. St Louis: The CV Mosby Company, 1993: 1119-51
4. Silver LB, editor. Learning disabilities. Child Adolesc Psychiatr Clin North Am 1993; 2
5. Duane DD. Learning disabilities. In: Frank Y, editor. Pediatric behavioral neurology. Boca Raton (Fl): CRC. In press
6. Sandler AD, Watson TE, Footo M, et al. Neurodevelopmental study of writing disorders in middle childhood. J Dev Behav Pediatr 1992; 13: 17-23

7. Critchly M. The dyslexic child. Springfield (Il): Charles C. Thomas, 1970
8. Orton ST. 'Word-blindedness' in school children. Arch Neurol Psychiatry 1925; 14: 581-615
9. Strauss AA, Lehtinen LE. Psychopathology and education in the brain-injured child. New York: Grune & Stratton, 1947
10. National Advisory Committee on Handicapped Children. Special education for handicapped children. Washington (DC): Department of Health, Education and Welfare, 1968
11. American Psychiatric Association. Diagnostic and statistical manual of mental disorders. 4th ed. Washington, DC: American Psychiatric Association, 1994
12. Hynd GW, Cohen M. Dyslexia: neuropsychological theory, research, and clinical differentiation. New York: Grune & Stratton, 1983
13. Rutter M. Prevalence and types of dyslexia. In: Benton AL, Pearl D, editors. Dyslexia, an appraisal of current knowledge. New York: Oxford University Press, 1978: 3-28
14. Rutter M, Yule W. The concept of specific reading retardation. J Child Psychol Psychiatry 1975; 16: 181-97
15. Shaywitz SE, Shaywitz BA, Fletcher JM, et al. Prevalence of reading disability in boys and girls: results of the Connecticut longitudinal study. JAMA 1990; 264: 998-1002
16. DeFries JC. Gender ratios in reading-disabled children and their affected relatives: a commentary. J Learn Disabil 1989; 22: 544-55
17. Strang JD, Rourke BP. Arithmetic disability subtypes: the neuropsychological significance of specific arithmetic impairment in childhood. In: Rourke BP, editor. Neuropsychology of learning disabilities: essentials of subtype analysis. New York: Guilford Press, 1985: 167-83
18. Bruck M. Persistance of dyslexics' phonological awareness deficits. Dev Psychol 1992; 28: 874-86
19. Stiles-Davis J. Spatial dysfunctions in young children with right hemisphere injury. In: Stiles-Davis J, Kritchevsky M, editors. Spatial cognition brain bases and development. Hillsdale (NJ): Lawrence Erlbaum, 1988: 251-72
20. Rourke BP. Nonverbal learning disabilities. The syndrome and the model. New York: Guilford Press, 1989
21. Stuss DT, Benson DF. The frontal lobes. New York: Raven Press, 1986
22. Goldman-Rakic PS. Circuitry of primate prefrontal cortex and regulation of behavior by representational knowledge. In: Plum F, editor. Handbook of physiology. Section 1: The nervous system. Vol. 5. Higher functions of the brain. New York: Oxford University Press, 1987: 373-417
23. Eliason MJ. Neurofibromatosis: implications for learning and behavior. Dev Behav Pediatr 1986; 7: 175-9
24. Welsh MC, Penington BF, Ozonoff S, et al. Neuropsychology of early-treated phenylketonuria: specific executive function deficits. Child Dev 1990; 61: 1697-713
25. Bellinger DC, Needleman HL. Lead and the relationship between maternal and child intelligence. J Pediatr 1983; 102: 523-7
26. Needleman HL, Bellinger D, Leviton A. Does lead at low dose affect intelligence in children? Pediatrics 1981; 68: 894-6
27. Bender BH, Puch M, Salenblatt J, et al. Cognitive development of children with sex chromosome abnormalities. In: Smith S, editor. Genetics and learning disabilities. San Diego: College Hill Press, 1987: 175-201
28. Galaburda AM. The testosterone hypothesis: reassessment since Geschwind and Benan. Ann Dyslex 1990; 40: 18-38
29. Galaburda AM. Neurology of developmental dyslexia. Curr Opin Neurol Neurosurg 1992; 5: 71-6
30. Scarborough H. Prediction of reading disability from familial and individual differences. J Educ Psychol 1989; 81: 101-8
31. Thomas W. Congenital 'word blindness' and its treatment. Ophthalmoscope 1905; 3: 380-3
32. Hinshelwood J. Four cases of congenital word-blindness occurring in the same family. BMJ 1907; 2: 1229-32
33. Finucci JM, Guthrie JT, Childs AL, et al. The genetics of specific reading disability. Ann Hum Genet 1976; 40: 1-23
34. Penington BF, Gilger JW, Pauls D, et al. Evidence for major gene transmission of developmental dyslexia. JAMA 1991; 266: 1527-34
35. Smith SD, Pennington BF, Kimberling WJ, et al. Familial dyslexia: use of genetic linkage data to define subtypes. J Am Acad Child Adolesc Psychiatry 1990; 29: 204-13
36. Olson R, Wise B, Conners F, et al. Specific deficits in component reading and language skills: genetic and environmental influences. J Learn Disabil 1989; 22: 339-48
37. Smith SD, Kimberling WJ, Penington BF, et al. Specific reading disability. Identification of an inherited form through linkage analysis. Science 1983; 219: 1345-7
38. Cardon LR, Smith SD, Fulker DW, et al. Quantitative trait locus for reading disability on chromosome 6. Science 1994; 266: 276-9
39. Lambert NM, Sandoval J. The prevalence of learning disabilities in a sample of children considered hyperactive. J Abnorm Child Psychol 1980; 8: 33-50
40. Silver L. The relationship between learning disabilities, hyperactivity, distractibility, and behavioral problems. J Am Acad Child Psychiatry 1981; 20: 385-97
41. Anderson JC, Williams S, McGee R, et al. DSM-III disorders in preadolescent children. Arch Gen Psychiatry 1987; 44: 69-76
42. Denckla MB. Academic and extracurricular aspects of nonverbal learning disabilities. Psychiatr Ann 1991; 21: 717-24
43. Geschwind N, Levitsky W. Human brain: left-right asymmetries in the temporal speech region. Science 1968; 161: 186-7
44. Wittelson SF, Pallie W. Left hemisphere specialization for language in the newborn: neuroanatomical evidence of asymmetry. Brain 1993; 96: 641-6
45. Chi JG, Dooling EC, Gilles FH. Left-right asymmetry of the temporal speech areas of the human fetus. Arch Neurol 1977; 34: 346-8
46. Galaburda AM. Dyslexia: a neurologic update. Neurol Chron 1993; 2: 1-5

47. Sherman GF, Galaburda AM, Geschwind N. Cortical anomalies in brains of New Zealand mice: a neuropathologic model of dyslexia? Proc Natl Acad Sci USA 1985; 82: 8072-4
48. Humphreys P, Rosen GD, Press DM, et al. Freezing lesions of the developing rat brain. A model for cerebrocortical microgyria. J Neuropathol Exp Neurol 1991; 50: 145-60
49. Denckla MB, LeMay M, Chapman CA. Few CT scan abnormalities found even in neurologically impaired learning disabled children. J Learn Disabil 1985; 18: 132-5
50. Hynd GW, Sermud-Clikeman M, Lorys AR, et al. Brain morphology in developmental dyslexia and attention deficit disorder/hyperactivity. Arch Neurol 1990; 47: 919-26
51. Duara R, Kushch A, Gross-Glen K, et al. Neuroanatomic differences between dyslexic and normal readers on magnetic resonance imaging scans. Arch Neurol 1991; 48: 410-6
52. Leonard CM, Voeller KS, Lombardino LJ, et al. Anomalous cerebral morphology in dyslexia revealed with magnetic resonance imaging. Arch Neurol 1993; 50: 461-9
53. Gross-Glenn K, Duara R, Barker WW, et al. Positron emission tomographic studies during serial word-reading by normal and dyslexic adults. J Clin Exp Neuropsychol 1991; 13 (4): 531-44
54. Hagman JO, Wood F, Buchsbaum MS, et al. Cerebral brain metabolism in adult dyslexic subjects assessed with positron emission tomography during performance of an auditory task. Arch Neurol 1992; 42: 734-9
54a. Shaywitz SE, Shaywitz BA, Puch KR, et al. Functional disruption in the organization of the brain for reading in dyslexia. Proc Natl Acad Sci USA 1998; 95: 2635-41
55. Duffy FH, Denckla MB, Bartels PH, et al. Dyslexia: regional differences in brain electrical activity by topographic mapping. Ann Neurol 1980; 7: 412-20
56. Landwehrmeyer B, Gerling J, Wallesch CW. Patterns of task-related slow brain potentials in dyslexia. Arch Neurol 1990; 47: 791-7
57. Kingsbourne M. Learning disabilities. In: Vinken PJ, Brayn GW, Klawans HL, editors. Handbook of clinical neurology. Rev. series 2. Vol. 46. Neurobehavioral disorders. Amsterdam: Elsevier Science Publishers, 1985: 123-37
58. Frank Y, Seiden JA, Napolitano B. Event related potentials to an 'oddball' auditory paradigm in children with learning disabilities with or without attention deficit hyperactivity disorder. Clin Electroencephalogr 1994; 25: 136-41
59. Livingstone MS, Rosen GD, Drislane FW, et al. Physiological and anatomical evidence for a magnocellular defect in developmental dyslexia. Proc Natl Acad Sci USA 1991; 88: 7943-7
60. Galaburda AM, Corsiglia J, Rosen GD, et al. Planum temporale asymmetry. Reappraisal since Geschwind and Levitsky. Neuropsychologia 1987; 25: 853-68
61. Galaburda AM, Aboitiz F, Rosen GD, et al. Histological asymmetry in the primary visual cortex of the rat: implications for mechanisms of cerebral asymmetry. Cortex 1986; 22: 151-60
62. Duane DD. The medical and neurological diagnostic process in learning disabilities. Child Adolesc Psychiatr Clin North Am 1993; 2: 283-93
63. Denckla MB. Revised neurological examination for subtle signs. Psychopharmacology 1985; 21: 773-99
64. Lovett MW. Developmental dyslexia. In: Segalowitz SJ, Rapin I, editors. Handbook of neuropsychology. Vol 7: child neuropsychology. Amsterdam: Elsevier Science Publishers, 1992: 163-85
65. Scarborough H. Very early language deficits in dyslexic children. Child Dev 1990; 61: 1728-43
66. Pennington BF, Van Orden G, Smith SD, et al. Phonological processing skills and deficits in adult dyslexics. Child Dev 1990; 61: 1753-78
67. Mattis S, French JH, Rapin I. Dyslexia in children and young adults: three independent neuropsychological syndromes. Dev Med Child Neurol 1975; 17: 150-63
68. Kovacs M, Goldston D. Cognitive and social cognitive development of depressed children and adolescents. J Am Acad Child Adolesc Psychiatry 1991; 30: 388-92
69. Silver L. Psychological and family problems associated with learning disabilities: assessment and intervention. J Am Acad Child Adolesc Psychiatry 1989; 3: 319-25
70. Wise B, Olson RK. Remediating reading disabilities. In: Obrzut JE, Hynd GW, editors. Advances in the neuropsychology of learning disabilities: issues, methods, and practice. New York: Academic Press, 1991
71. Lerner JW. Educational interventions in learning disabilities. J Am Acad Child Adolesc Psychiatry 1989; 28: 326-30
72. Runyan MK. The effect of extra time on reading comprehension scores for university students with and without disabilities. In: Shaywitz SE, Shaywitz BA, editors. Attention deficit disorder comes of age: towards the twenty-first century. Austin (TX): PRO-ED, 1992: 185-95
73. Hagin R, Silver A. Learning disorders in childhood. New York: Wiley, 1990
74. Wolkowitz OM, Tinkelburg JR, Weingartner H. A psychobiological perspective of cognitive functions. Neuropsychobiology 1985; 14: 88-96
75. Schneider LS, Olin JT. Overview of clinical trials of hydergine in dementia. Arch Neurol 1994; 51: 787-98
76. Rozzini R, Zanetti O, Bianchetti A. Treatment of cognitive impairment secondary to degenerative dementia. Effectiveness of oxiracetam therapy. Acta Neurol (Napoli) 1993; 15 (1): 44-52
77. Gallai V, Mazzotta G, Del Gatto F. A clinical and neurophysiological trial on nootropic drugs in patients with mental decline. Acta Neurol (Napoli) 1991; 13 (1): 1-12
78. Di Ianni M, Wilsher CR, Blank MS. The effects of piracetam in children with dyslexia. J Clin Psychopharmacol 1985; 5: 272-8
79. Wilsher CR, Bennett D, Chase CH. Piracetam and dyslexia: effects on reading tests. J Clin Psychopharmacol 1987; 7: 230-7

80. Ackerman PT, Dykman RA, Holloway C, et al. A trial of piracetam in two subgroups of students with dyslexia enrolled in summer tutoring. J Learn Disabil 1991; 24 (9): 542-9
81. Rapoport JL, Buchsbaum MS, Weingartner H, et al. Dextroamphetamine: cognitive and behavioral effects in normal and hyperactive boys and normal men. Arch Gen Psychiatry 1980; 37: 933-43
82. Abikoff H, Gittelman R. The normalizing effects of methylphenidate on the classroom behavior of ADHD children. J Abnorm Child Psychol 1985; 13: 33-4
83. Greenhill LL. Attention deficit hyperactivity disorder. The stimulants. Child Adolesc Psychiatr North Am 1995; 4: 123-68
84. Wilens TE, Biederman J. The stimulants. Psychiatr Clin North Am 1992; 15: 191-222
85. Dulcan M. Using psychostimulants to treat behavior disorders of children and adolescents. J Child Adolesc Psychopharmacol 1990; 1: 7-20
86. Birmaher BB, Greenhill LL, Cooper MA. Sustained release methylphenidate: pharmacokinetic studies in ADHD males. J Am Acad Child Adolesc Psychiatry 1989; 28: 768-72
87. Carlson CL, Thomeer ML. Effects of ritalin on arithmetic tasks. In: Greenhill LL, Osman B, editors. Ritalin: theory and patient management. New York: Mary Ann Liebert, 1991: 195-202
88. Sprague RL, Sleator EK. Methylphenidate in hyperkinetic children: differences in dose effects on learning and social behavior. Science 1977; 198: 1274-6
89. Sallee F, Stiller R, Perel J. Pharmacodynamics of pemoline in attention deficit disorder with hyperactivity. J Am Acad Child Adolesc Psychiatry 1992; 31: 244-51
90. Hunt RD, Capper L, O'Connell P. Clonidine in child and adolescent psychiatry. J Child Adolesc Psychopharmacol 1990; 1: 87-102
91. Biederman J, Gastfriend DR, Jellinek MS. Desipramine in the treatment of children with attention deficit disorder. J Clin Psychopharmacol 1986; 6: 359-63
92. Biederman J, Baldessarini RJ, Wright V, et al. A double-blind placebo controlled study of desipramine in the treatment of ADD. II: Serum drug levels and cardiovascular findings. J Am Acad Child Adolesc Psychiatry 1989; 28: 903-11
93. Biederman J, Baldessarini RJ, Wright V, et al. A double-blind placebo controlled study of desipramine in the treatment of ADD. I: Efficacy. J Am Acad Child Adolesc Psychiatry 1989; 28: 777-84
94. Gualtieri CT, Keenan PA, Chandler M. Clinical and neuropsychological effect on desipramine in children with attention deficit hyperactivity disorder. J Clin Psychopharmacol 1991; 11: 155-9
95. Satz P, Taylor G, Friel J, et al. Some developmental and predictive precursors of reading disabilities: a six-year follow-up. In: Benton AL, Pearl D, editors. Dyslexia: an appraisal of current knowledge. New York: Oxford University Press, 1978: 315-47
96. Rourke BP, Orr RR. Prediction of the reading and spelling performances of normal and retarded readers: a four-year follow-up. J Abnorm Child Psychol 1977; 5: 9-20
97. Schonhaut S, Satz P. Prognosis for children with learning disabilities. A review of follow-up studies. In: Rutter M, editor. Developmental neuropsychiatry. New York: Guilford Press, 1983: 542-63
98. Apree O. Prognosis of learning disability. J Consult Clin Psychol 1988; 56: 836-41
99. Baker L, Cantwell DP. A prospective psychiatric follow-up of children with speech/language disorders. J Am Acad Child Adolesc Psychiatry 1987; 26: 546-53
100. Bender WN. Secondary personality and behavioral problems in adolescents with learning disabilities. J Learn Disabil 1987; 20: 280-5
101. Silver LB. The misunderstood child: a guide for parents of children with learning disabilities. 2nd ed. New York: McGraw-Hill, 1992
102. What happens next? Trends in postschool outcomes of youth with disabilities. The second comprehensive report from the National Longitudinal Transition Study of Special Education Students. Office of Special Education Programs. US Department of Education. SRI International, 1992 Dec: 6-32-6-36

Correspondence: Dr *Yitzchak Frank,* Division of Pediatric Neurology, Departments of Neurology and Pediatrics, North Shore University Hospital, Cornell University Medical College, 300 Community Drive, Manhasset, NY 11030, USA.

Gilles de la Tourette's Syndrome
A Guide to Pharmacological Treatment

Lisbeth Regeur,[1] Lene Werdelin,[1] Henning Pakkenberg[2] and Rasmus Fog[3]

1 Department of Neurology, Bispebjerg Hospital, Copenhagen, Denmark
2 Neurological Research Laboratory, Bartholin Instituttet, Kommunehospitalet, Copenhagen, Denmark
3 St. Hans Hospital, Department P, Roskilde, Denmark

1. Clinical Features

Gilles de la Tourette's syndrome (TS) is a neuropsychiatric disorder characterised by involuntary motor and vocal tics, and associated with a variety of behavioural disturbances (see table I). Previously, patients with this syndrome were rarely diagnosed. However, since the first reports of effective treatment of symptoms of the syndrome with haloperidol in 1961[1-2] recognition of this disorder has improved, and recent epidemiological studies indicate that TS is no longer rare.[3]

During the last two decades, research into the genetic, neurophysiological, neurochemical, neuropharmacological and neurobehavioural mechanisms of TS has intensified, and important advances have been made. Recent research has suggested that TS may be inherited by autosomal dominant transmission.[4,5] However, attempts to localise the responsible gene have not yielded consistent results thus far, and recently alternative models have been proposed (for review see Robertson[3]). Furthermore, family studies provide support for a common genetic basis for TS and some forms of obsessive-compulsive symptoms.[6,7] A genetic relationship between TS and attention deficit hyperactivity disorder (ADHD) has also been proposed.[8] However, it remains to be clarified which of these associated behavioural problems are intrinsic to TS and which simply have a frequent comorbidity.[9-11] Recently an association between group A β-hemolytic streptococcal infections and the development of tics, TS and obsessive-compulsive disorder (OCD) has been reported by several groups. A possible role of postinfectious immune-mediated mechanisms in the pathogenesis of TS has been suggested.[3,12,13]

Since the essential pathophysiology of TS is still not known and many attempts to demonstrate neurotransmitter changes have been inconsistent,[14,15] some of the best clues for further understanding the neurochemical pathology of the disorder are derived from pharma-

Table I. Behavioural disorders associated with Gilles de la Tourette's syndrome

Obsessive-compulsive disorder
Attention deficit hyperactivity disorder
Conduct disorders
Learning disabilities
Depression
Anxiety

cological experience. The strong effect of antidopaminergic agents on motor and vocal tics in TS led to the ical hypothesis of a dopaminergic hyperactivity in the basal ganglia.[16] However, the variety of medications capable of suppressing tics and other features of TS has led to the suggestion that other neurotransmitters, such as noradrenaline (norepinephrine), serotonin (5-hydroxytryptamine; 5-HT), γ-aminobutyric acid (GABA), acetylcholine and opioids, are also involved.[17,18] This has been the basis for alternative treatment strategies.

2. Pharmacological Treatment

Pharmacological treatment, which is the only proven effective treatment for motor and vocal symptoms of TS, is strictly symptomatic and should be directed primarily at reducing tic symptoms. The decision to initiate drug therapy is based on the severity of motor and vocal tics and their potential for adversely affecting the psychosocial, educational and occupational functioning of the patient.

Treatment is unnecessary if symptoms are mild and do not interfere with psychosocial functioning. In patients in whom tic symptoms are functionally disabling, the goal of treatment is to reduce tics to a tolerable level with the lowest possible drug dosage.[17,18] The optimal dosage has to be individually titrated to achieve maximum effectiveness with minimal adverse effects. Numerous drugs have been used in the treatment of TS with different degrees of effect. In the following sections, some of the most frequently used drugs will be discussed.

2.1 Antidopaminergic Drugs

At present, drugs that block central dopaminergic neurotransmission are the most effective in suppressing tic symptoms in TS.

2.1.1 Haloperidol

Haloperidol is a butyrophenone antipsychotic agent that binds more specifically to post-synaptic dopamine D_2 than to D_1 receptors. It also has some α_1-adrenergic antagonistic activity. The drug was first used to treat TS in 1961[1,2] and was subsequently reported to improve symptoms in 62 to 91% of patients.[10,19,20] As a result, it was soon considered the drug of choice. Unfortunately, frequent adverse effects, such as sedation, dysphoria, bodyweight gain, movement abnormalities (bradykinesia, akathisia, acute dystonic reactions), depression, poor school performance and school phobias, limit the usefulness of this medication even at low doses.[17,21,22] Furthermore, 9 cases of haloperidol-induced tardive dyskinesias have been reported in the literature (see review by Shapiro[10]). However, none of the more than 3000 patients treated by Shapiro[10] developed tardive dyskinesias, probably because of the low dosage used. Because of the adverse effects of haloperidol other agents with similar therapeutic action, but with fewer adverse effects, have been investigated, such as pimozide.

2.1.2 Pimozide

Pimozide is a diphenylbutylpiperidine. Like haloperidol it preferentially binds to D_2 receptors, but has little effect on adrenergic receptors. Pimozide is equipotent with haloperidol in treating TS,[23] but in several trials of other hyperkinetic diseases it was shown to have fewer adverse effects.[24,25]

Since 1979, pimozide has been the drug of choice in our treatment of TS. This is because of the impression that the drug induces fewer adverse effects and so is better tolerated that haloperidol. This view is also shared by other groups.[17,22,23] However, there is no firm evidence that pimozide is more effective than other antipsychotics. In a trial of pimozide involving 65 patients, a good response was found in 73% and a moderate response (with adverse effects not necessitating discontinuation or reduction of dosage) in a further 9% of patients with dosages up to 8 mg/day.[26] Most of the patients experienced transient sedation in the first weeks of treatment. Other adverse effects encountered in pimozide-treated patients were body-weight gain, depression, pseudo-Parkinsonism and akathisia. We did not see acute dystonia or tardive dyskinesia, probably because of low dosages and slow increments of dosage increase. In only very few patients, anticholinergics were needed to treat the adverse effects.

Prolongation of the QT interval has been reported with pimozide, and related to the calcium channel blocking properties of the drug.[10,27] Furthermore, sinus bradycardia has been reported with the combination of fluoxetine and pimozide.[28] If QT interval is abnormal on the initial electrocardiogram (ECG), pimozide should be avoided. Thus, in our experience, pimozide is as effective as haloperidol and has fewer adverse effects.

2.1.3 Tetrabenazine

In some patients, the therapeutic effect of pimozide decreases with time. In such cases and if adverse effects of pimozide become unacceptable, tetrabenazine should be considered as an alternative. Tetrabenazine, a benzoquinoline derivative that depletes presynaptic storage of monoamines, has been found to be effective in a variety of hyperkinetic movement disorders, including TS.[29,30] Although tetrabenazine can induce acute dystonic reactions, no case of tardive dyskinesia has been documented with this drug. In a cohort of 65 patients, 10 were treated with tetrabenazine in dosages from 25 to 100 mg/day with good or moderate response.[26] Adverse effects observed were drowsiness and depression, while Parkinsonian adverse effects were not seen in this dosage range. In 5 of the patients, tetrabenazine at dosages ranging from 25 to 50 mg/day was combined with pimozide (1 to 8 mg/day) because of adverse effects or a decreased effect of tetrabenazine. By combining two antidopaminergic agents with different sites of action, a more lasting effect with fewer adverse effects was obtained at lower dosages of each drug.

2.1.4 Alternative Antidopaminergic Drugs

In patients not responding to pimozide, tetrabenazine or haloperidol, other antipsychotic drugs should be tried.

In several studies, fluphenazine, a piperazine phenothiazine, has been reported to be as effective as haloperidol, but to be associated with fewer adverse effects when administered at daily dosages of 2 to 15mg.[14,31,32] The type of adverse effects seen are the same as with other antidopaminergic drugs, with the exception of a lower frequency of sedation.

Sulpiride is a substituted benzamide with selective D_2 receptor blocking effects that has been extensively used by some groups.[3] It is associated with a lower incidence of adverse effects than classical antipsychotics, particularly extrapyramidal adverse effects and sedation. However, it is associated with some adverse effects, principally bodyweight gain and gynecomastia. The drug was successfully tried in a few patients alone or in combination with pimozide in dosages ranging from 100 to 400 mg/day.

Risperidone, a benzisoxazole, is one of the new atypical antipsychotic drugs with potent $5-HT_2$ and D_2 receptor blocking properties. In dosages of 1 to 6 mg/day the drug appears to have a lower risk of extrapyramidal adverse effects when compared with traditional antipsychotics. It may be an interesting alternative especially in patients with TS and OCD. In several open-label trials, a beneficial effect on TS symptoms has been reported. However, one group found the effect somewhat disappointing (for review see Robertson[3]). The most common adverse effects reported were sedation, bodyweight gain, akathisia, dystonic reactions, galactorrhoea and dysphoric mood.[33]

In a recent trial, ziprasidone, another new atypical antipsychotic drug with $5-HT_2$, and D_2 receptor blocking and $5-HT_{1A}$ receptor agonistic effects, was significantly more effective than placebo in reducing tics in 28 patients with TS in dosages ranging from 5 to 40 mg/day.[34] Mild transient somnolence but no extrapyramidal adverse effects were seen. It was concluded that ziprasidone offers an alternative to available therapies for the treatment of TS. However, further studies are necessary to evaluate its safety and efficacy.

Olanzapine, a $5-HT_2$, D_2 and D_1 receptor antagonist, has recently been reported to be effective in one case of severe TS.[35]

2.2 Noradrenergic-Modulating Drugs

Pharmacological studies with clonidine have suggested that noradrenergic mechanisms are involved in the pathophysiology of TS. Clonidine, an imidazole derivative, is an adrenergic agonist that in low doses diminishes central noradrenergic activity by stimulating presynaptic α_2-adrenergic autoreceptors, thus inhibiting the release of noradrenaline. In several studies, it has been reported to relieve motor tics, vocalisations and behavioural symptoms in at least 50% of patients.[31,36,37] As a result some groups consider clonidine to be the drug of first choice for children with TS and ADHD.[3]

When used in TS the initial dosage should be very low, e.g. 0.025 mg/day. The dosage should be slowly increased over several weeks to a maximum of 0.3 mg/day. Adverse effects include sedation (often transient) which occurs in about 30% of recipients, and dizziness, dry mouth, headaches and depression in 10 to 30% of patients. Discontinuation should be gradual to avoid hypertensive rebound. In patients with associated behavioural symptoms, we have used clonidine in dosages of 0.1 to 0.225 mg/day with moderate effect. When combined with pimozide, a good clinical response on both motor tics and behavioural symptoms was obtained in these patients.[26]

Clonidine transdermal patches have also been used. Using this formulation, Comings[38] obtained improvement in 60% of over 300 patients in terms of both tics and behavioural symptoms. Adverse effects were sedation and skin irritation.

Guanfacine, a more recently developed α_2-adrenergic agonist that appears to be less sedating and hypotensive than clonidine, has been reported to be beneficial in the treatment of both ADHD and TS.[39]

2.3 Serotonin Reuptake Inhibitors

The associated behavioural symptoms in TS (OCD, ADHD and conduct disorders) are often less improved by antipsychotics than are the tic symptoms. Previously, if these symptoms predominated and seriously interfered with social functioning, a treatment protocol would have been to combine an antipsychotic with clonidine. During the last two decades, however, the pharmacotherapy of OCD has been revolutionised by the development of potent serotonin reuptake inhibitors.[38,40]

2.3.1 Clomipramine

Clomipramine, a tricyclic antidepressant that strongly inhibits serotonin reuptake, has been the most extensively studied agent in OCD. Complete suppression or marked improvement of symptoms in 50% of patients has been reported.[41] We have used clomipramine in some of our patients with associated behavioural symptoms starting with 25 mg/day and up to a maximum of 150 mg/day. We observed a good clinical response on behavioural symptoms in at least 50% of patients. The tic symptoms most often necessitated combination treatment with antipsychotics (e.g. pimozide). Adverse effects within these dose limits were minor and included sedation, dry mouth and constipation. Children may be at greater risk of the cardiotoxic effects of tricyclic antidepressants than adults.[40,42] Therefore, treatment with these agents must be preceded by a baseline ECG assessment.

2.3.2 Selective Serotonin Reuptake Inhibitors

Agents such as citalopram, fluoxetine, fluvoxamine, paroxetine and sertraline belong to a new generation of antidepressants; the selective serotonin reuptake inhibitors (SSRIs). They have very little affinity for dopaminergic, noradrenergic and cholinergic receptors. Unlike the tricyclic antidepressants they are not cardiotoxic, and they have minimal anticholinergic adverse effects. All have been found to be well tolerated and effective in the treatment of OCD.[43]

Fluoxetine, the first clinically available SSRI, has been shown to be very effective in many patients with TS.[38] In a double-blind, placebo-controlled trial, 50% of patients showed substantial improvement of obsessive-compulsive symptoms while receiving fluoxetine 10 to 40 mg/day.[44] We have used citalopram and fluoxetine 20 to 60 mg/day and sertraline 50 to 150 mg/day in many of our patients. A significant improvement in behavioural symptoms, but less effect on motor tics, was observed.

Coadministration of an SSRI and pimozide has been found to result in a good clinical response and an enhancement of the anti-obsessional effect of the SSRI (unpublished observations). A similar effect was previously reported with a combination of fluvoxamine and pimozide.[45] There were few adverse effects of this combination, and those that did occur included nervousness, transient insomnia, transient nausea, and restlessness. Combinations with other dopamine antagonists such as sulpiride and haloperidol have also been reported.[3,43]

2.4 Tricyclic Antidepressants

Whereas the SSRIs are often very effective in the treatment of the obsessive-compulsive symptoms in TS they seem less effective than tricyclic antidepressants in the treatment of ADHD. Imipramine, a tricyclic agent that is a less potent serotonin reuptake inhibitor than clomipramine, is suggested in these patients in dosages of 25 to 75 mg/day, as it is less likely to cause or increase motor tics than psychostimulants (see section 2.4). As mentioned in section 2.3.1, there is a risk of cardiotoxic effects and, therefore, treatment with imipramine and other tricyclic antidepressants should be preceded by baseline ECG assessment.

Nortriptyline has recently been shown to be effective for the symptoms of ADHD in the presence of tics, and could be used as an alternative to imipramine.[46]

2.5 Psychostimulants

Components of ADHD are present in 50 to 80% of children with TS.[17,38] Psychostimulants [e.g. methylphenidate, dexamphetamine (dextroamphetamine) and pemoline] are the drugs of choice for the treatment of children with ADHD.[11] In the treatment of ADHD in patients with TS, the use of psychostimulants has, however, been controversial since they may precipitate or exacerbate tics in 20 to 25% of the patients.[3,11,47,48] We, therefore, currently recommend treatment with clonidine or antidepressants combined with pimozide. If these drugs are ineffective, a trial with methylphenidate 2.5 to 10 mg/day should be initiated. If tics are not worsened, the treatment may be maintained at dosages of 15 to 30 mg/day together with pimozide 2 to 6 mg/day. Other groups, however, recommend treatment of ADHD in TS with methylphenidate as the first drug of choice.[10,11,38]

2.6 Alternative Agents

Not all patients benefit from treatment with antipsychotics or the other treatment strategies mentioned in sections 2.2, 2.3, 2.4 and 2.5. In some patients, treatment has to be stopped because of intolerable adverse effects. Various agents with different mechanisms of action have been recommended in these patients, including clonazepam,[49] lithium,[31] carbamazepine,[38] baclofen,[38] cholinergic drugs (e.g. physostigmine),[50] opioid antagonists[51] and calcium channel blockers.[52] Furthermore, in a few patients, we have used vigabatrin, an antiepileptic drug that specifically inhibits GABA transaminase. This agent has some beneficial effect on motor tics (unpublished observations).

Lamotrigine blocks voltage-dependent sodium channels and probably acts by preventing the release of excitatory neurotransmitters, predominantly glutamate. We have used it in 3 patients. At a dosage of 400 mg/day, this treatment has in 1 patient resulted in a substantial reduction of motor and vocal tics and behavioural problems for more than 7 years. In the other 2 patients treatment was abandoned because of skin rash (1) and lack of effect (1).

Different dopamine agonists have been used. In an open trial selegiline (deprenyl), a selective monoamine oxidase-B inhibitor, was reported to improve ADHD in 90% of 29 patients with TS.[53] In a later controlled trial there was no statistically beneficial effect of selegilinel on ADHD symptoms, but a marginal effect on motor tics.[54]

Recently, small doses of pergolide, a mixed D_1-D_2-D_3 receptor agonist, has been reported to significantly improve symptoms in children with TS. The presence of restless leg comorbidity was highly associated with a positive response.[55,56]

Botulinum toxin is now increasingly used by several groups in the treatment of focal dystonic and vocal tics.[57,58]

The efficacy of all these alternative drugs remains questionable and requires further investigation.

3. Treatment Strategies

Drug treatment should only be started in patients with TS who have functionally disabling symptoms. Table II summarises the agents that can be used.

For tics our drug of first choice is pimozide. We start with doses of 0.5 to 1 mg/day and increase the dosage by 0.5 to 1 mg/day every seventh day. It may be an advantage to give the drug twice daily (morning and afternoon) since in many patients the greatest reduction in symptoms is associated with peak plasma drug concentrations. Our maximum dose is normally 8 mg/day. The limiting factor with pimozide is adverse effects. The optimal effect is normally a 70% reduction of symptoms without adverse effects.

Table II. Agents for the treatment of Gilles de la Tourette's syndrome

Drug[a]	Dosage (mg/day)		Adverse effects
	starting	maximum	
Antidopaminergic agents			
Fluphenazine	0.5	10	Similar to other antidopaminergic agents, lower incidence of sedation
Haloperidol	0.25	6-8	Sedation, dysphoria, bodyweight gain, bradykinesia, akathisia, acute dystonia, tardive dyskinesias, depression, poor school performance, school phobias
Pimozide	0.5-1	8	Bodyweight gain, depression, pseudo-Parkinsonism, akathisia, prolongation of QT interval
Sulpiride	100	400	Bodyweight gain, gynecomastia
Tetrabenazine	12.5	100	Drowsiness, depression
Serotonin reuptake inhibitors			
Citalopram	10-20	60	Nervousness, insomnia, headache, nausea, sexual disturbances
Clomipramine	25	150	Cardiotoxicity (obtain an electrocardiogram before starting treatment), dry mouth, constipation, sedation, sexual disturbances
Fluoxetine	10-20	60	Nausea, nervousness, insomnia, headache, sexual disturbances
Fluvoxamine	25-50	150	Nausea, constipation, agitation, insomnia, sexual disturbances
Paroxetine	10-20	60	Nausea, sweating, tremor, insomnia, sexual disturbances
Sertraline	50	200	Nausea, diarrhoea, sweating, tremor, somnolence, sexual disturbances
Stimulants			
Dexamphetamine	5	30	Decreased appetite, insomnia, irritability, exacerbation of tics
Methylphenidate	2.5-10	30	Decreased appetite, insomnia, irritability, exacerbation of tics
Other agents			
Clonidine	0.025	0.3	Sedation, dizziness, dry mouth, headaches, depression
Flunarizine[b]	1	10	Depression, headache, bodyweight gain
Lamotrigine[b]	25	600	Rash, dizziness, ataxia, somnolence
Vigabatrin[b]	1000	4000	Sedation, irritability, headache, psychoses
Selegiline (deprenyl)	5	10	Nausea, agitation, irritability, drowsiness, headache, diarrhoea, tic exacerbation
Pergolide	0.025	0.3	Sedation, dizziness, nausea, stomach ache, irritability, exacerbation of ADHD

a   Agents can be used in combination, e.g. pimozide and sulpiride.

b   Can be used in patients nonresponsive to or unable to tolerate other agents.

ADHD = attention deficit hyperactivity disorder.

If the effect with pimozide is insufficient our next step is to change to tetrabenazine. We start with a dosage of 12.5 mg/day and gradually increase the dosage by 12.5mg every seventh day to a maximum of 100 mg/day. If the effect is poor, we try a combination of pimozide and tetrabenazine. If the treatment outcome still is unsatisfying, clonidine is substituted for tetrabenazine. The clonidine dosages should be low, starting with 0.025 mg/day and gradually increased to 0.3 mg/day.

There are great individual differences in the response to drugs. This means that if the above-mentioned standard regimen is not successful we change the medication to other antipsychotics. The order is generally: haloperidol (0.25 mg/day, up to a maximum of 6 to 8 mg/day), fluphenazine (0.5 mg/day, up to a maximum of 8 mg/day) and sulpiride (100 mg/day, up to a maximum of 400 mg/day). Some of these agents can also be tried in combination. A pimozide-sulpiride combination in low dosages (e.g. 2 to 6 mg/day and 100 to 400 mg/day, respectively) has shown beneficial effects in some patients (unpublished observations)

The treatment regimen has to be individualised. The patients should learn to adjust the dosage according to the severity of symptoms and, if possible, to taper off medication in periods with few symptoms. A strict regimen with low dosages, which is often possible with combinations of drugs with different mechanisms of action, and small and gradual changes of dosages are the best ways to avoid long term adverse effects, such as tardive dyskinesia.

If behavioural problems such as OCD, anxiety or depression are disabling we start with a selective serotonin reuptake inhibitor. We use citalopram or fluoxetine in dosages of 10 mg/day increasing to a maximum of 40 to 60 mg/day or sertraline starting at 50mg/day increasing to 150 mg/day. The drugs are most often used as add-on to pimozide. In the case of a poor response, we change to clomipramine 25 mg/day, slowly increasing to a maximum of 150 mg/day. In cases of disabling ADHD problems or conduct disorder, we use clonidine or, alternatively, we combine pimozide with clonidine.

In patients with severe ADHD, a trial with stimulants may be attempted. Recommended starting dose is 2.5 to 10 mg in the morning. If symptoms improve and tics are not exacerbated, the dosage, if necessary, can be gradually increased to a maximum of 30 mg/day. In patients who fail to respond to treatment, we try flunarizine up to 10 mg/day, vigabatrin (up to 4000 mg/day) or lamotrigine (slowly increased up to 300 mg/day) – all in combination with pimozide.

In patients with sleep-initiating problems, clonidine at a single dose of 0.1 to 0.2mg or the hormone melatonin can be helpful.

4. Conclusion

Strategies for managing the full spectrum of TS often involve several classes of medication to obtain optimal therapy. Although the number of medications to treat TS patients has increased, adverse effects are still a major problem. More effective therapeutic agents with fewer adverse effects are still needed.

Acknowledgements

The authors wish to thank Dr. Bente Pakkenberg for a fruitful and very inspiring collaboration.

References

1. Seignot MJN. Un cas de maladie des tics de Gilles de la Tourette gueri par le R-1625. Ann Med Psychol 1961; 119: 578-9
2. Caprini G, Melotti V. Un grave sindrome ticcosa guerita con haloperidol. Riv Sper Freniat 1961; 85: 191-6
3. Robertson MM. Invited review. Tourette syndrome, associated conditions and the complexities of treatment. Brain 2000; 123: 425-62
4. Kurlan R, Behr J, Medved L, et al. Familial Tourette's syndrome: report of a large pedigree and potential for linkage analysis. Neurology 1986; 36: 772-6
5. Curtis D, Robertson MM, Gurling HM. Autosomal dominant gene transmission in a large kindred with gilles de la Tourette syndrome. Br J Psychiatry 1992; 160: 845-9
6. Robertson MM. The Gilles de la Tourette syndrome: the current status. Brit J Psychiatry 1989; 154: 147-69
7. Robertson MM. The relationship between Gilles de la Tourette's syndrome and obsessive compulsive disorder. J Serotonin Res 1995; Suppl. 1: 49-62
8. Knell ER, Comings DE. Tourette's syndrome and attention-deficit hyperactivity disorder: evidence for a genetic relationship. J Clin Psychiatry 1993; 54: 331-7
9. Bruun RD, Budman CL. The natural history of Tourette syndrome. In: Chase TN, Friedhoff AJ, Cohen DJ, editors. Tourette syndrome: genetics, neurobiology, and treatment. New York: Raven Press, 1992: 1-6
10. Shapiro AK, Shapiro E. Neuroleptic drugs. In: Kurlan R, editor. Handbook of Tourette's syndrome and related tic and behavioral disorders. New York: Marcel Dekker, Inc., 1993: 347-75
11. Freeman RD. Attention deficit hyperactivity disorder in the presence of Tourette syndrome. Neurol Clin 1997; 15: 411-20
12. Swedo SE, Leonhard HL, Garvey M, et al. Pediatric autoimmune neuropsychiatric disorders associated with streptococcal infections: clinical description of the first 50 cases. Am J Psychiatry 1998; 155: 264-71
13. Kurlan R. Tourette's syndrome and 'PANDAS': will the relation bear out? Neurology 1998; 50: 1530-4
14. Jankovic J. The neurology of tics. In: Marsden CD, Fahn S, editors. Movement disorders 2. London: Butterworths, 1987: 383-405
15. Robertson MM, Stern JS. Tic disorders: new developments in Tourette syndrome and related disorders. Curr Opin Neurol 1998; 11: 373-80
16. Snyder SH, Taylor KM, Coyle JL, et al. The role of brain dopamine in behavioural regulation and the actions of psychotropic drugs. Am J Psychiatry 1970; 127: 199-207
17. Singer HS, Walkup JT. Tourette syndrome and other tic disorders: diagnosis, pathophysiology, and treatment. Medicine 1991; 70: 15-32
18. Singer HS. Neurobiology of Tourette syndrome: review. Neurol Clin 1997; 15: 357-79
19. Shapiro AK, Shapiro E, Wayne H, et al. Treatment of Tourette's syndrome with haloperidol, review of 34 cases. Arch Gen Psychiatry 1973; 28: 92-7
20. Shapiro AK, Shapiro ES, Bruun RD, et al. Gilles de la Tourette syndrome. 2nd ed. New York: Raven Press, 1988
21. Bruun RD. Subtle and underrecognized side effects of neuroleptic treatment in children with Tourette's disorder. Am J Psychiatry 1988; 145: 621-4
22. Salee FR, Nesbitt L, Jackson C, et al. Relative effect of Pimocide in children and adolescents with TS. Am J Psychiatry 1997; 154: 1057-62
23. Ross MS, Moldofsky H. A comparison of pimozide and haloperidol in the treatment of Gilles de la Tourette's syndrome. Am J Psychiatry 1978; 135: 585-7
24. Pakkenberg H, Fog R. Spontaneous oral facial dyskinesia: results of treatment with tetrabenazine, pimozide or both. Arch Neurol 1974; 31: 352-3
25. Fog R, Pakkenberg H. Theoretical and clinical aspects of the Tourette syndrome (chronic multiple tic). J Neural Transm 1980; Suppl. 16: 211-5
26. Regeur L, Pakkenberg B, Fog R, et al. Clinical features and long-term treatment with pimozide in 65 patients with Gilles de la Tourette's syndrome. J Neurol Neurosurg Psychiatry 1986; 49: 791-5
27. Fulop G, Phillips RA, Shapiro AK, et al. ECG changes during haloperidol and pimozide treatment of Tourette's disorder. Am J Psychiatry 1987; 144: 673-5
28. Ahmed I, Dagincourt PG, Miller LG, et al. Possible interaction between fluoxetine and Pimozide causing sinus bradycardia. Can J Psychiatry 1993; 38: 62-3
29. Pakkenberg H. The effect of tetrabenazine in some hyperkinetic syndromes. Acta Neurol Scand 1968; 44: 391-3
30. Jankovic J, Beach J. Long-term effects of tetrabenazine in hyperkinetic movement disorders. Neurology 1997; 48: 358-62
31. Borison RL, Ang L, Chang S, et al. New pharmacological approaches in the treatment of Tourette syndrome. In: Friedhoff AJ, Chase TN, editors. Gilles de la Tourette Syndrome. New York: Raven Press, 1982: 377-82
32. Goetz CG, Tanner CM, Klawans HL. Fluphenazine and multifocal tic disorders. Arch Neurol 1984; 41: 271-2
33. Bruun RD, Buchman CL. Risperidone as treatment for Tourette's syndrome. J Clin Psychiatry 1996; 57: 29-31
34. Salee FR, Kurlan R, Goetz CG, et al. Ziprasidone treatment of children and adolescents with Tourette's syndrome: a pilot study. J Am Acad Child Adolesc Psychiatry 2000; 39: 292-9
35. Bhadrinath BR. Olanzapine in Tourette syndrome [letter]. Br J Psychiatry 1998; 172: 366
36. Cohen DJ, Detlor J, Young JG, et al. Clonidine ameliorates Gilles de la Tourette syndrome. Arch Gen Psychiatry 1980; 37: 1350-7
37. Leckman JF, Hardin MT, Riddle MA, et al. Clonidine treatment of Gilles de la Tourette's syndrome. Arch Gen Psychiatry 1991; 48: 324-8
38. Comings DE. Tourette syndrome and human behavior. California: Hope Press, 1990

39. Chappell PB, Riddle MA, Scahill LS, et al. Guanfacine treatment of comorbid attention-deficit hyperactivity disorder in Tourette's syndrome: preliminary clinical experience. J Am Acad Child Adolesc Psychiatry 1995; 34: 1140-6
40. King RA, Riddle MA, Goodman WK. Psychopharmacology of obsessive-compulsive disorder in Tourette syndrome. In: Chase TN, Friedhoff AJ, Cohen DJ, editors. Tourette syndrome: genetics, neurobiology, and treatment. New York: Raven Press, 1992: 283-91
41. Leonard HL, Swedo SE, Rapoport JL, et al. Treatment of obsessive-compulsive disorder with clomipramine and desipramine in children and adolescents: a double-blind crossover comparison. Arch Gen Psychiatry 1989; 46: 1088-92
42. Riddle MA, Nelson JC, Kleinman CS, et al. Sudden death in children receiving Norpramin: a review of three reported cases and commentary. J Am Acad Child Adolesc Psychiatry 1991; 30: 104-8
43. Rapoport JL, Inoft-Germain G. Medical and surgical treatment of obsessive-compulsive disorder. Neurol Clin 1997; 15: 421-8
44. Riddle MA, Scahill LS, King RA, et al. Double-blind, crossover trial of fluoxetine and placebo in children and adolescents with obsessive-compulsive disorder. J Am Acad Child Adolesc Psychiatry 1992; 32: 1062-9
45. McDougle CJ, Goodman WK, Price LH, et al. Neuroleptic addition in fluvoxamine-refractory obsessive-compulsive disorder. Am J Psychiatry 1990; 147: 652-4
46. Spencer T, Biederman J, Wilens T, et al. Nortriptylin treatment of children with attention-deficit hyperactivity disorder and tic disorder or Tourette's syndrome. J Am Acad Child Adolesc Psychiatry 1993; 32: 205-10
47. Price RA, Leckman JF, Pauls DL, et al. Gilles de la Tourette's syndrome: tics and central nervous system stimulants in twins and nontwins. Neurology 1986; 36: 232-7
48. Robertson MM, Eapen V. Pharmacological controversy of CNS stimulants in Gilles de la tourette's syndrome. Clin Neuropharmacol 1992; 15: 408-25
49. Truong DD, Bressman S, Shale H, et al. Clonazepam, haloperidol, and clonidine in tic disorders. South Med J 1988; 81: 1103-5
50. Stahl SM, Berger PA. Physostigmine in Tourette syndrome: evidence for cholinergic underactivity. Am J Psychiatry 1981; 138: 240-2
51. Sandyk R. The effects of naloxone in Tourette's syndrome. Ann Neurol 1985; 18: 367-8
52. Micheli F, Gatto M, Lekhuniec E, et al. Treatment of Tourette's syndrome with calcium antagonists. Clin Neuropharmacol 1990; 13: 77-83
53. Jankovic J. Deprenyl in attention deficit associated with Tourette's syndrome. Arch Neurol 1993; 50: 286-8
54. Feigin A, Kurlan R, McDermott MP, et al. A controlled trial of deprenyl in children with Tourette's syndrome and attention deficit hyperactivity disorder. Neurology 1996; 46: 965-8
55. Lipinski JF, Sallee FR, Jackson C, et al. Dopamine agonist treatment of Tourette disorder in children: results of an open-label trial of pergolide. Mov Disord 1997; 12: 402-7
56. Gilbert DL, Sethuraman G, Sine L, et al. Tourette's syndrome improvement with pergolide in a randomized, double-blind, crossover trial. Neurology 2000; 54: 1310-5
57. Jankovic J. Botulinum toxin in the treatment of dystonic tics. Mov Disord 1994; 9: 347-9
58. Trimble MR, Whurr R, Brookes G, et al. Vocal tics in Gilles de la Tourette syndrome treated with botulinum toxin injections. Mov Disord 1998; 13: 617-9

Correspondence: Dr *Lisbeth Regeur*, Department of Neurology, Bispebjerg Hospital, DK-2400 Copenhagen NV, Denmark.